MAYBE
THEY LEFT
TOOLS
IN MY
BRAIN

MAYBE THEY LEFT TOOLS IN MY BRAIN

BY JONATHAN MILLER

ISBN: 978-1-7376305-0-0
Ebook ISBN: 978-1-7376305-1-7

Manufactured in the United States of America.
Produced by Dean Burrell.
Design by Maureen Forys, Happenstance Type-O-Rama.
Cover Design by Randy McKee.

10 9 8 7 6 5 4 3 2 1

www.enterstageleft.com

To all of the survivors, professionals, and caregivers out there who have inspired me to navigate this course of recovery in one way or another, I am eternally grateful.

ACKNOWLEDGMENTS

Somehow, I've always been blessed with surrounding myself with great people. For me to mention everyone who has impacted my life over the course of these forty years or this specific journey in any capacity would be borderline impossible. You all know who you are.

CONTENTS

CONTENTS

PREFACE

T he following pages are based on events mainly from my memory, personal journal entries, and recounts of medical processes explained by professionals, colleagues, and family at times when my judgment may have been compromised by medical events. A few names have been changed to protect the identity of those who wish to remain anonymous. I'd say it's pretty darn spot on, however likely not perfect. After all, I had brain surgery—what's your excuse?

Without giving away too much of the plot in the pages that follow, you'll likely realize that music has played a huge role in my life over the years. The result of the hemorrhagic stroke left me with severe paralysis on the left side of my body. As a result, my ability to play guitar was stripped from me. In the ensuing months, I also learned that a small piece of my vocal chord that affected my range was impacted. These were devastating blows on several levels, as the reality slowly set in that the recovery process was far more intricate than I had originally expected. Each chapter's title pays homage to the bands and musicians who have molded me throughout the years. There was no intended agenda to pair a song with any particular event in my life, yet I found patterns beginning to form and small vignettes were seemingly created.

So, if you choose to dig a little deeper into my musical palette, feel free to dig up these gold sounds as you see fit. I'm not going to spoon-feed you the sauce, but you'll figure out the formula. Now, without further ado, what do you say we start the show!

1

RANDOM RULES

When I landed my first actual sales position in February of 2003, I had no clue as to what I was getting into. When you combine any sort of entry-level sales interview process with a not-fully-developed adolescent brain, the functionality of making clear career decisions sometimes becomes rather skewed, to say the least. Every smart manager has the same bullshit rags-to-riches tales in their arsenal of how, "if you work really hard in your first three months you'll be in line to hit your first base salary raise, and furthermore, if you work your ass off within the first year, you'll be making six figures and get promoted to manager," yada, yada.

And trust me when I say that I fell into the trap more than once as I started to navigate through the whole struggle as a young professional. I've been suckered into selling watercooler systems in Center City Philadelphia, hawking Cutco knives, trying to pass the

LAH exam to be licensed to sell health insurance (thank Christ that was a bust), even trying my hand at retail, pushing cell phones at the Granite Run Mall (God rest its soul) in a last-ditch effort not to have to accept defeat. No matter what it took to simply stay afloat, I was not retreating back to central Pennsylvania.

I was parked on a side street in Newark, Delaware, grinding through another dreadful, soaking wet day of business-to-business cold calling trying to pitch any and every mom-and-pop car dealership, dry cleaner, nail spa, convenience store cashier, barbershop proprietor, tarot card reading establishment, and bowling alley concession stand attendant as to why they needed to invest in purified spring water and the time is now. And it was the same pitch each time, to take advantage of this deal now because of this "onetime-only opportunity" that I was offering on this particular day. I was becoming bored, frustrated, impatient, and then downright bitter. Then my tiny Nokia cell phone (remember those little numbers that revolutionized the cellular phone call experience back in the day?) started buzzing with one of those lackluster yet catchy tunes that stick inside your head forever. A guy named Doug Donohoe introduced himself from the other side of the line about yet another sales representative position opening in Middlesex, New Jersey. I had submitted my resume to a handful of entry-level sales positions throughout Philadelphia and New Jersey. He stated that my resume had come across his desk and began his spiel that he and his business partner were currently looking for outside sales representatives for their franchise-based logistics outfit. In my typical expeditious manner, I responded that I was currently trying to hustle watercooler units for some pyramid-scheme, half-assed chop shop of a marketing company out of Philly, in which I was pretty close to throwing in the towel due to the simple misrepresentation of the product. He said something to the effect of, "Well, that's just what we're looking for up here, so I'd like to bring you in for an interview in the next week or so." I thought, "Of course, what can it hurt?" after listening for a few minutes of what the position entailed.

I didn't think too much of it once we lined up the particulars for a face-to-face interview.

As I crossed back across the PA border later that day, I started to reflect on the honest shelf life of slinging H2O carousels and delivery with no rhyme or reason to the approach of each day. I further started to ponder why eight out of ten peers with whom I started out four weeks prior had resigned formally or simply didn't show up the next day. The team faded out quickly. I finally figured out that lousy salespeople had sold me on an equally lousy sales opportunity. I quickly had the epiphany that this half-assed racket was not for me. I had a handful of sales that I was to be paid out on so I figured the right thing to do was to call the manager and tell her that I was finished, effective immediately. Then I would demand my commissions, which had accrued over the past six or seven weeks, be paid in the form of a check that I would personally pick up at the office during business hours. Something gave me the hunch that I'd never see those funds if I put the ball in their court, so I showed up unannounced a couple days later to personally collect my hard-earned compensation. That was a tough lesson learned in the world of multi-level marketing scams, let me tell you.

I still mention this story, in some way, in almost every interview that I have conducted throughout the years—the tale of how that one phone call changed the game for me. Obviously, I respectfully resigned from the water jug slinging position in the coming days with one thought in mind: "If I can survive six weeks selling watercooler systems door to door in central Philadelphia, I can survive just about anything!"

Anyway, I followed up with this Doug character after he gave me some insight into what his company did as a reseller channel for a large overnight shipping operation. The company was called Worldwide Express, headquartered in Dallas, Texas. Back then, Worldwide was a franchise-based, third-party overnight shipping outfit that had partnered with Airborne Express a decade earlier. Airborne was the low-cost shipping alternative to the duopoly of Federal Express and

UPS in the overnight shipping space. The founders of the company had brilliantly pitched Airborne executives about implementing an outside-sales-driven franchise model to specifically focus on small to medium-sized business. In providing low retail rates with localized customer service, the model would rapidly increase growth for their low-cost overnight shipping product. The concept proved to be successful, resulting in small offices of driven, entrepreneurial-spirited talent around the country. When I learned what their outside sales model was all about during the corporate training that was provided, it sounded a hell of a lot more appealing than hustling H2O around the "Badlands." Through the process of a couple interviews with Doug and his business partner, Leon, followed by a field ride around the territory, I was offered the position on a Friday and accepted it the next Monday. I was pumped for the new opportunity, but also, it fell in line perfectly as my girlfriend had recently accepted a career advancement offer with a large cosmetic company she had interned with while studying logistics two years earlier. A few of our peers and mentors were biting their bottom lips thinking that we wouldn't survive for six months out there mainly due to an inflated cost of living, and the rest simply thought, "Screw it, why not? Godspeed!" Regardless, everything was lining up spectacularly; we signed off on an apartment lease and purchased a number of minimal furniture items. The moving excursion was made over the course of roughly eighteen hours in a delivery van that my uncle let us use. We turned right back around that evening after unloading and made a very drowsy voyage back to PA in the early hours of the morning. Everything else would be crammed into our own vehicles and hauled off across the border.

The first order of business after the ink dried for this new employment endeavor was to attend a five-day "basic sales training" seminar in Dallas, where the corporate office was located. There, a group of fifty or so "hungry for success, green behind the ears" trainees would be taught the basic strategies of effective business-to-business cold-call selling, how to line up a meeting with a true decision maker, and how to run through the "Seven Steps of the Sale," which were all taught by the executive vice president of sales who had the military training and leadership style of Stonewall Jackson. He was one of the most intense, passionate business personalities that I had ever met to that point. Those five days, cooped up in a swanky Hilton property surrounded by Dallas proper, were a complete whirlwind. The training was like a 300-level college course that sucked you up and spit you out—all wrapped up into one of the most intense weeks on record to that point in my life. I got so much out of the whole experience. I even got to hobnob with the CEO and COO, which, to my knowledge, were two of the wealthiest hands that I had ever shaken. The formality of the entire week had the grave undertone a young cadet would expect. "Look around, people; most of these faces will not be here a year from now," they would mutter.

Due to the intense schedule, I didn't have downtime to explore much of the city. Most of us were young and broke, so even with the per diems generously given by our ownership groups for food, transportation, and sundries, I (at least) didn't have much spare loot to get too adventurous. I do vividly remember Dallas being hot and flat, though. Very hot and very flat, and I asked myself, "Why would anyone ever want to live here?"

Honestly, I was more confused about what I had gotten myself into upon boarding that jet and leaving DFW International Airport than when I had arrived five days earlier. This regimen of an organization chewed us trainees up and regurgitated us back to our respective offices throughout the country, but I returned back to Jersey with a well-refined knowledge of the business and sales process. I did come to realize in the days immediately following that I had a few key details in my favor. Doug and Leon, for one. Their work-hard, play-hard mentality was very refreshing, and they were extremely plugged in to this business model. Not to mention, this company's culture was right up my alley.

2

HERE COMES A
REGULAR

Author's Note:

Allow me to pause here for a moment and explain that my intention throughout these writings is not to bog you, the reader, down with a pile of medical terminology, research findings, case studies, statistics, counter hypotheses, theory, or jargon. There are thousands upon thousands of books and publications that go into the minutiae of determining specific diagnoses and treatments based on research.

What I will give you is a glance into my personal journey of a series of compelling events that led to an intense rehabilitation process, which these years later, has seemed to metamorphose into a pretty amazing and interesting quality of life. To reflect on certain journal entries written (which I will be sharing with you to illustrate time frames and where my state of mind was) is to show the indescribable impact of a young person's life when medical situations of epic proportion hit unexpectedly.

This is one of the few terms that is extremely imperative to understand . . .

Aura: *A sensation perceived by a patient that precedes a condition affecting the brain. An aura often occurs before a migraine or seizure. It may consist of flashing lights, a gleam of light, blurred vision, an odor, the feeling of a breeze, numbness, weakness, or difficulty in speaking.*

* * *

As a teenager, then into my twenties, a realization set in. There had to be some way to connect my cranium to some sort of medical device that could read brain activity. And then, if a professional in the field of study could acutely interpret the results, one would notice that something out of the ordinary was going on up there when these episodes hit. The problem was that I never knew when they would fire and for how long. Well, shortly after the shit hit the fan, I found out that there indeed was a device that could detect seizure activity called an electroencephalogram (EEG), which tests for epileptic episodes. During an EEG screening, electrical signals from the brain are recorded by sensors placed on the individual's scalp. I had my first EEG evaluation done in Princeton, New Jersey, months after my surgery to determine if the activity was constant or intermittent. My aura episodes were typically intermittent, which was proven to be accurate once the neurologist viewed the results and explained the findings to us. The fact that I was epileptic was diagnosed immediately and accurately. The problem was that I wasn't totally honest with my doctors or my family regarding these episodes. I'd been dealing with this condition for so long that I thought I had it all under control. Episodes would occur that at times were very intense and at other times were rather euphoric. In a way, I wanted this to be my own little secret. Even though I was sure that these spasms were atypical, I kept this little internal demon to myself. I didn't want some unpronounceable medical title to be attached to the spells. I didn't know if this was good activity, bad activity, a neurological warning sign, or perhaps I was simply the Son of God.

My aura spells formed my earliest childhood memories, dating back to when I was four years old. One may think, "It would be almost impossible to retain that sort of vivid memory at that age." So, let me give you some validation. Those who know me well will typically affirm that my long-term memory is bizarrely precise and accurate. A quick example would be that I can give you a detail-by-detail account of an ice cream stand that we visited at the base of Pikes Peak in Manitou Springs, Colorado, when I was seven years old (including what flavor was chosen and the outfit I was wearing at the time), but I couldn't tell you accurately what I had for dinner three nights ago because it would take a certain degree of concentration and focus. Now, after I think of the setting, venue, and situation, it goes into a long-term memory bank, which gets played back and forth in my head multiple times then stored into a special vault of tens of thousands of clips and visually recorded moments of time that very seldom escape from my long-term memory factory.

A word of advice here is to not ever bet me on remembering past events unless you are 100 percent confident about what occurred. I very seldom lose wagers of this nature. It's how I somehow remember every lyric to every track in order from the Beastie Boys album *Licensed to Ill* put out by Def Jams Records in November of 1986 including a complete visual explanation of the artwork from the cassette sleeve right down to the specific area of the sleeve for which loyal fans could write in inquires "for T-shirts, and bullshit." Or how I know that Timothy McVeigh's favorite ice cream was mint chocolate chip and he asked for it as his last meal before he was executed via lethal injection for the Oklahoma City bombings (the ice cream theme is simply a coincidence). I've got a mental card catalog of random knowledge and fun facts of epic proportions. Even so, my brain functionality would likely not be a solid fit for competition on a show like *Jeopardy*, for example. Reason being that my mind chooses to completely embrace certain subject material such as music, art, space, history, pop culture, and geography but tends to shut out topics such as mathematics, politics, current events, literature, sports statistics, and modern-day television programs along with the celebrities who are cast in them.

Anyway, the first aura episode I remember distinctly happened when I was four years old. It occurred in my parents' bedroom on the far side of the room next to the queen-sized bed. I remember the bedspread with the red roses pattern, which I assume was a typical fashion style back then. The sensation crept up into my head in the exact same epileptic fashion as it enters to this day, in an intense and threatening trespass with little or no warning. It strangles my brain waves with the power of a boa constrictor and does not release until the intent is fulfilled. I physically stop and feel the event begin to take shape. I don't move. I only concentrate. It forms into a pattern of waves and sounds that pulsate and shift as the feeling sees fit. It is very sharp but painless, and I can never shake it out. The feeling is so vivid and intense. It always has a build, climax, and de-crescendo, which can be frightening and aggressive or complex and twisted. I used to sometimes think it was relaxing with a slight sense of euphoria. But that was all before I understood that the aura is a warning signal that precedes the possible seizure activity. Twenty-four years later, I lived the reality.

The episodes are always different in feeling, intensity, and experience, but these storms typically roll in and exit the same. It was the feeling when I gave Jessica Dodson one last kiss after the last bell rang and school let out in ninth grade when we finally decided to break up for good. As soon as I boarded bus #63 and took a seat beside a member of my crew, an aura episode ripped through my head for the entire bus ride home. I sat there bracing myself as the episode took shape from the weight of the "seismic" event that manifested itself moments before. Or, the time that my buddy Jamie (Chuck) Chestney found a way to score us tickets for the Nine Inch Nails/David Bowie concert in Pittsburgh when I was a senior in high school and I was overwhelmed with excitement and anticipation. Or, at my high school graduation months later where I literally had a session of brain activity that lasted for the entire commencement at Mansion Park in May of 1996. And even a few years back at my annual Worldwide Express sales conference in Fort Lauderdale after a bender of a celebration when our office hit our projected sales numbers, I would spend an incredible evening drenched in booze, wine, and heavy petting with a female executive from our corporate office in her posh hotel suite overlooking the Atlantic Ocean. When I was ready to leave her room at six thirty the following morning, I was gathering my necktie and suit jacket when an episode of aura ripped through my head with an impact of a punch to the skull. And it was the explosion that attacked my head the exact same way when I hit the River Road entrance ramp to Route 18 in Piscataway, New Jersey, on February 19, 2006, as I pegged the gas pedal to the floor of my 530i to merge into the sea of erratic lunchtime traffic. In a few moments, my entire life would be impacted to a degree of immense proportion. And this would start the cascade of events that I am sharing with you now.

Journal Entry: November 17, 2006

An event was going to happen that would change my life. My body and strength would be taken away. All that remained was my damaged brain, heart, and soul. It was my job to heal myself. I would build myself back from a wheelchair and a hospital bed. I would learn a great deal and speak of the triumph. This is how I want it written when the time comes.

3

GROOVE IS IN
THE HEART

grew up in the rural town of Altoona, Pennsylvania, located roughly
120 miles east of Pittsburgh. With a population of 44,000 people, it
still bears the decrepit skeleton of a major staging area for the Pennsylvania rail line in the middle of the nineteenth century expanding
travel between Pittsburgh and Philadelphia. As major corporations
started to gobble up smaller entities of the PRR and B&O railroading
companies and pensioned workers were eventually retired off and
fizzled out, the corporations that moved in brought their own management and labor styles, and naturally, the railroad industry slowed
as faster and more lucrative forms of travel expanded.

I always had a fairly neutral outlook on where I grew up. Granted,
my neighborhood was an amazing dynamic of middle-class roots,

where many decided to raise their families as well, which is how Bellmeade Drive became such a blast of an environment to grow up in. My grandparents built their homestead off of that road in the fifties. My parents decided to raise my two sisters and me in that very house, and several of my friends fell into the same formula as well. Our dads were all friends growing up, and my gang of "Bellmeade Boys" still remains an extremely close unit to this day. Most neighborhoods that I've come across don't seem to have the same repeat of generational pass-down as ours did. Sure, there were so many of us that cliques and brotherhood societies formed depending on interests and athletic ability. As we grew up, several families on that three-mile stretch of road molded and shaped us into the "bright, upstanding role models of character that we are today" (or something like that). No matter if we went to the same schools, were in the same grade, or rode the same bus, you could typically locate the swarms of us playing baseball, football, damming a stream, building tree stand structures, riding bikes, or looting the local Sheetz convenience store or Best Way Pizza at the end of our street. Our parents didn't seem to worry about our whereabouts either because there was always an activity to be had. I never had a curfew. I don't think any of us did growing up.

Anyway, I was a pretty straitlaced kid when it came to schooling. Sure, I was a polite nose-picking yap, so to speak, with multiple forms of lousy '80s haircuts resting upon a big-eared, scrawny, underweight frame. Teachers pointed out that I was polite and respected authority, which were likely the traits of a proper upbringing. I was considered a bit of a class clown back then, caring far more about making people laugh or rolling their eyes in disbelief at the simple shenanigans that I would pull off than taking my pursuit of academic achievements seriously. I never belonged to any particular social clique either. I wasn't a jock but was an avid skier, snowboarder, and tennis player. I wasn't a punk but loved the Sex Pistols and Primus. I wasn't studious in the least, but I thoroughly enjoyed History, English, Science, and the arts (so long as I had an inspiring teacher). I didn't run around with a mischievous crew, but I wasn't a saint. You get the point. If I thought someone had an interesting personality or hobbies, I would engage them. Otherwise, I was constantly with the other Bellmeade clowns engaging in acts of typical male adolescent horseplay in a world that seemed so secure.

Allow me to break away again to make one statement perfectly clear: I was in no way studious in those days, nor did I give a shit! I did not adhere to the concept of public education in the least. I had multiple teachers with whom I did not see eye to eye. However, just as I'm indebted to the handful of tremendous doctors, PTs, OTs, and speech pathologists who had the patience to take a holistic approach to my recovery later in life, so, too, am I grateful to the couple handfuls of teachers and professors who motivated and inspired me back in the day.

Learning in a classroom setting was a challenge for me back then. Terms such as ADD and ADHD were still very taboo, especially for mothers of children who weren't making classroom progress. I struggled with this throughout the majority of my academic career. As competitive and problem solving in nature as my personality is today, all I intended to achieve academically in grade school was to keep my head above water each year. Even if a teacher or professional had brought a laundry list of examples of my struggles to my mother, she would have certainly rejected a diagnosis of ADD or ADHD immediately. The crazy part is—even back then, I knew there was a problem.

Author's Note:

And yes, I get it. I find it amazing that virtually everybody is "terrible at math." Everyone says they are bad at math. It becomes an absurd statement. Even brilliant engineers, astrophysicists, and mathematicians say the same stupid line every time: "Yeah, I really was never that good at math." Well, here is what I say: "Shut up, you pompous clowns!" You want to see "bad at math," come hang out with me on a Saturday afternoon. The sheer act of figuring out the gratuity on a

$58.00 bar tab gives me an unexplainable sense of intense anxiety to this day. I can't explain it. And don't tell me about all that "move the decimal place over one space to figure out 10 percent" horseshit either! It simply doesn't compute. My brain is not wired in a mathematical fashion. The results of my senior-year SAT scores provide evidence of this. And to give credit where credit is due on this subject, I had a few teachers who spent several hours trying to make my brain understand how the puzzle pieces fit to the formulas of basic algebra and geometry alike. I also must give a shout-out to my mother who spent a lot of money and travel time in balancing tutors and early-morning drives to school so I could get extra help. My mother told me years later that she lost nights of sleep fearing that I wouldn't pass my algebra requirements in my junior high and high school years. Funny, I had several restless nights fretting about the same issue.

And again I need to break off here to bring up a significant observation from a twitter post, which gained some well-deserved traction at some point in 2019 from a national news story. Granted, I have very little social media presence to date, but I think this particular tweet hit the nail on the head when it comes to educational views as seen by a multitude of Americans today. Quote: "It's 2019 . . . Get rid of Algebra 2 in high schools and replace it with Finance Fundamentals. Teach kids about careers (not just college), salaries, credit, budgeting, money management, taking out a loan, buying a house, filing their taxes." Brilliantly stated in less than 280 characters if I do say so myself!

* * *

So, to say that I was a B student academically at best is not far from an exaggeration. One of my preschool teachers characterized me as "The Absent-Minded Professor" at age five, which to this day explains a lot as to the way that I approach life. I was given an obscurely quirky and creative mindset, which may be a blessing or a curse depending on which way you want to look at it. In no way was I engaged in learning from a textbook standpoint. That was out! I'd much rather devise a fantastic ploy into how to sucker a gullible grandparent into buying me a random band's cassette or *Hit Parader* magazine, so I could learn about bands such as AC/DC, Aerosmith, Skid Row, Motley Crue, or Guns N' Roses. I wanted to learn about rock and roll icons and their lifestyles as well as artistic expression. My view back then was that mastering multiplication tables and spelling words was in no way necessary (and as we now see, my foresight was on-point as we type and text with autocorrect activated at all times, case closed!). Rather, my thought process was to learn just enough to make it look like I was semi-engaged in my studies. If my quarterly report cards would look mediocre to the parental eye (we all knew back then that a degree in nuclear physics was not going to be in my future), I should be able to skate under the radar for the remainder of elementary school to junior high so long as no "slacker red flags" came up, as that would then get my parents involved.

Allow me to give you an example of one of my roundabout, grand-plotted, reverse-psychology maneuvers to buck the sixth-grade system. Let's just say that my teacher that year, Mr. Fanelli, and I saw eye to eye on practically nothing. Yes, I was a bit of a class heckler back then. However, there was a bigger issue brewing. I was falling behind in my homework assignments (because the subject matter bored me), and, in essence, my grades—especially in math and spelling—began to suffer as well.

When you're twelve years old, your views of your academic fate are of no substance. I kept trying to explain to my parents that my teacher was completely disengaged from me. This bonehead's approach to "teaching" was a complete joke. He didn't like me for whatever reason and I didn't care for his bullshit one bit either. My folks shrugged it off and gave me an aggressive explanation as to why my sixth-grade year was so important—I was entering junior high school the following year, etc., etc., etc. So here was the strategy that I devised to a) get my grades up to an average range and b) teach this screwball a lesson about mind power and control.

A few of my Bellmeade crew (most of whom were more academically disciplined than I) were also in my class, and I knew that if I managed to sit close to one of my fellow cronies, they'd likely permit me to sneak a few glances at their homework and quizzes. Mr. Fanelli had us switch our desk assignments around after each marking period and I knew that I needed to get my marks up somehow or I'd surely be faced with the consequence of getting my parents involved. His method to the new desk assignment exercise was—he would arrange all names in a hat lottery system of sorts and begin drawing names front to back among the seven rows in the classroom. My theory was that I had enough of my buddies on my side that surely I'd get a desk position close to at least one of them. So, at the beginning of the third marking period, the day came when we drew our new seating assignments. As each name was drawn, I tactfully started to scope the room in a somewhat nervous, somewhat optimistic, somewhat praying state of anticipation.

And, of course, when my name was finally selected, I found myself nowhere even remotely close to any of my comrades. I felt a sense of nausea begin to set into my gut for a few seconds until the next name was read (this would be the desk occupied directly behind me for all intents and purposes). And . . . jackpot! This was an even better set of circumstances! Kimberly, my "girlfriend" of a month or something to that point, was now directly behind me. I had no clue at the time as to how this would all play out from an academic petty fraud scenario, mind you, but surely this girl would be a great resource (at least from a homework plagiarism standpoint). And for the first week or so, my theory was coming to fruition. My little girlfriend was more than happy to hand over her prior night's assignments for me to glance at and scribble fiercely for five minutes or so until Old Fanelli called the classroom to some sort of order. So, this part of my devised scheme was off to a brilliant start. That was . . . until our first pop quiz hit. Kimberly was behind me, which would serve as no help from a cheating standpoint, and my peers to my direct right and left were of no greater academic intelligence than I.

Soon after, the whole problem became dramatically clear and the demise rapidly began to take shape. Since I had Kimberly as a go-to homework source, I was now completing the absolute bare minimum of my homework, which naturally led to retaining the bare minimum of the subject matter as well. My homework was submitted 95 percent complete and furthermore correct, but my class marks were suffering because I had only minimal in-class knowledge of the materials. "Shit!" I thought. "The gig is going to come to a screeching halt if he catches on."

Did I mention that I was also a real chatterbox back then? Did I mention that Kimberly also loved Guns N' Roses? So, do you remember that *Hit Parader* magazine? Did I mention it contained a full spread on the *Appetite for Destruction* album, which was purchased by my completely oblivious grandfather in a time where schools and churches were educating parents that MTV content and heavy metal music were poisoning the youth of America? Well, the news of this publication—which I had acquired that weekend—rapidly swept from our Bellmeade Drive bus stop to the back of the bus, the jam-packed school lobby, and on into the classroom almost as quickly as the news that my buddy's *Sports Illustrated* 1989 swimsuit issue featuring Elle Macpherson on the cover had also made it onto the bucket of bolts and into the institute of educational excellence. When the news of my weekend score got to Kimberly, with a cute little glisten in her eye and a decisive nod, she knew exactly how to get her meat hooks onto this little anarchist's gem. She was more than willing to hand me her math worksheets on that particular Monday morning.

Now herein again lies the problem. Old Fanelli knew that I was up to some sort of mischief or plot right off the bat, partly because I'd pulled this sort of stunt before. If I remember correctly, I got busted sneaking Big League Chew onto the bus (not a big deal), then onto the school grounds via backpack (slightly bigger deal), and then the pouch made it to my jeans front pocket where the rat caught me nonchalantly gnawing on a few strands right before lunch. He forced me to throw my contraband in the garbage. But, as far as the magazine went, I think the main tip-off was that a bunch of my peers had already formed a huddle around me and started an aggressive barter campaign haggling tater tots, portions of lunch money funds, candy bars, and free chocolate milks to get a look at the pictures and articles at some point during the day. The issue now was that I had already given the magazine back to Kimberly to square away the homework transaction. I needed to make good on a couple of handshake deal promises before the end of the day and now my little friend didn't want to give back the goods. So, every five minutes, I would turn around in an attempt to compromise. I could tell that Fanelli was catching on to my disruptive jabber. However, if I didn't make true to my "clients," I knew that I was likely going to be heckled by my peers! Finally, as his back was turned and he began jotting something on the blackboard, he slammed the chalk down and turned around. The classroom was silent! Fanelli didn't say a word. Rather, he made this stupid nose wrinkle face, pointed at me, then pointed beside his desk. I was completely confused as to what he was instructing me to do. Within a second, a tingle came to my stomach and I understood as he motioned again. I was to pick up my desk and move it beside his. I was slightly humiliated but more so furious about the magazine at that moment.

The positive was that my magazine never got confiscated and he likely never figured out what all of the fuss and hype was about. Old Fanelli lectured me in the hall during the day's final bathroom break about how being disruptive like that was uncalled for and my new seating arrangement would be permanent until I showed signs of being more respectful of the classroom setting. At that moment, I wanted to rat out Kimberly and tell him that she held property of mine at ransom for no good reason. Perhaps this would get me off the hook. But I didn't say a word. After class was over and the busses pulled in to scoop us up, Kimberly came up to me and apologized for the whole thing as she gave me back my *Hit Parader* magazine. I think she knew that our little courtship was over due to the day's actions, but I told her that everything was all right. I appreciated the apology and enjoyed her friendship for several years to come.

Author's Note:

Now, back to Fanelli for a minute to finish this tale . . . For two weeks or so, my diminutive desk was placed right beside his. At least he didn't go as far as to get my parents involved; I surely would have taken a hot ass whipping from my father. Anyway, now that Kimberly was out of the equation regarding homework, I needed to shift my strategy to somehow keep my marks up. Well, I can tell you how Fanelli had made the stupidest decision affecting my elementary school career by throwing my seat next to his. First off, each morning right before the reciting of the pledge of allegiance, all written homework had to be submitted into a little plastic bin on his desk, which just happened to reside about a foot next to my new real estate. Within about two days, I realized the basket was like having your own plagiarizer's paradise at arm's reach so long as I was unassuming in my scheme. It worked like a charm! Even tests and quizzes were dropped into that bin upon completion as well. Are you kidding me? I mean, I knew fully well how the order of operations worked at the front of that classroom, but hardly knew how easy this would be to pull off! I started to jot small notes down on book covers of accessories that my gifted overachieving peers were wearing at the beginning of each morning so I could further coordinate my moves in a timely manner. I'd pay mind to any specific Swatch watch, pair of Nike AIR Jordan scuff marks from our flag football team, a color coded pair of Benetton socks, or specific jelly bracelet combinations that would catch my peripheral vision. Then, I'd strike like a viper once I knew the coast was clear. I'd managed to hit gold on this punishment that was now twisted completely upside down. Every minute that Fanelli's head was hunkered down devising lesson plans, grading papers, or when he was out in the hallway gossiping with other faculty, my eyes would gently gravitate up and to the right. At times I was nearly three feet from his face and he never had a clue. And what happened some weeks later? My class-room improvement was off the charts. I even made the Honor Roll that marking period just by figuring out a strategy to win at the game.

As a side note, as I reflect on the above . . . I never got a thrill out of cheating in this fashion; I just knew that I had to survive this educational punishment. Those years of elementary school were beyond frustrating. I acted out quite a bit and didn't think it would become any easier as I pushed ahead either.

4

SUBTERRANEAN HOMESICK ALIEN

F ebruary 17, 2006, began as a typical Friday. About a year earlier, Christy and I had socked away enough dough to purchase
our first home, which was a little gem in Milltown, New Jersey.
We bought a small yet swanky two-bedroom unit in a complex of
about twenty brownstone-like townhomes. The industrial-like complex boasted oversized front room windows, exposed original brick
and beams on both floors, and great views of Washington Avenue
from the third and fourth stories.

The alarm was on point for a five forty-five wake-up call. I'd
watch a little local news (paying mind to traffic and weather reports),
shower, pick a shirt/tie/dress pant/belt/shoe combo that fit the day
properly, chat with Christy about what our respective days looked

like, probably speak of loose dinner plans (it was a Friday and all). After finishing up in the bathroom, my wife would give a thumbs-up or adjust my tie, tell me to "have a great day," and we'd exchange kisses. I would then always put my dress shoes on at the top of the wooden stairs exiting the master bedroom leading down the narrow staircase to the living room and kitchen, seldom ingesting breakfast and never drinking coffee. Yes, you heard that one correctly—to this day, I have never had a sip of coffee in my life. Trust me, I have the personality of a coked-up Jack Russell terrier as it is, so no caffeine perk needed in this system. I was finally out the door by 6:50. The office was eight miles away and the commute typically took forty to fifty minutes depending on local traffic congestion and my rash New Jersey driving habits, which naturally kicked in after two years of commuting in the Garden State. Those fifty minutes or so were a great part of my typical workday. I'd usually be catching up with friends, family, or coworkers on the phone while toggling between terrestrial radio stations such as K-Rock, tuning in to hear what Howard and the FCC were bickering about; NJ 101.5, listening to passive talk radio while receiving current traffic updates; or WPRB Princeton ("Sponsored in part by the Princeton Record Exchange!"), which is how I discovered the enchanted melodies of the Pixies, Pavement, Built to Spill, The White Stripes, The Replacements, The Velvet Underground, and Uncle Tupelo. The key was to hit rush-hour traffic on Easton Avenue and I287 just right, which would put me at the office by quarter to eight to get my day organized. I had brought on three sales representatives a few months ago, and as sales manager, that meant that my days were often jam packed trying to juggle these new jockeys while simultaneously trying to stay updated with my senior sales crew, key account representatives, my bosses, and office administration personnel.

This particular morning was going to be interesting because I had back-to-back obligations with two of my rookies' reps meeting, my boy, Kevin in the northwest part of the territory at ten followed by a one o'clock in the southern part of our market with Michael.

The issue here was trying to slip through New Brunswick before I got pinned in the lunch rush traffic. Both guys knew that this day was going to be a beating from a logistical standpoint but certainly doable. Kevin and I ran the meeting, de-briefed in the parking lot for five minutes, and I told him that we would catch up once I got back to the office at the end of the day. I got in my car and looked at my watch. Pretty good shape, I thought! I had just over an hour to get down to East Brunswick to meet Mike. I hit the gas and combatively bolted down Route 202 toward Interstate 287, then jumped off at the River Road exit to cut across and head south on Route 18. Not five minutes into the drive, I hit my first situation. On 287 southbound, traffic was heavy. I felt my chest begin to tighten because there was nothing that I could do besides bounce back and forth between lanes while creeping along at a snail's pace. I popped a random compact disc into the player, then called Mike to give him my coordinates and ETA—at this point, I knew that I would be cutting it pretty close. I ended the call and began to spit a plethora of vulgar language at the traffic blocking my path. There were neither police nor emergency vehicles in sight. "Where the fuck is this traffic coming from?" I roared, while grinding my teeth and switching over to the radio to pick up a traffic report off of NJ101.5.

One of my largest gripes on the planet is tardiness for anything of importance. My entire team knew my policy on being punctual for just about everything on my calendar. I seldom broke this rule for myself unless it was a matter of dire concern. I clinched the steering wheel tight. Finally, after ten dreadful minutes, the crawling vehicles started to pick up momentum. I reacted accordingly, weaving and swerving around the more lethargic vehicle operators traveling at less than tolerable speeds. I finally hit the River Road exit. At this point I was in a semi-panicked state knowing all the while that, due to high levels of vehicle congestion from Rutgers University and the Johnson and Johnson corporate offices, the traffic situation on the next stretch of the journey very well might put me in the same bottleneck. To make matters worse, the idiots who had engineered the road back in the day put one completely out-of-place traffic light on Commercial Avenue, which backed up the traffic flow something awful.

I catapulted off of the exit at speeds that at any other time would be borderline erratic and reckless. This three-mile stretch was my only chance to shave off time as I bullishly blew through intersections along the Raritan River. I finally could see the Landing Lane street sign, immediately followed by the Rutgers football stadium to my left. I was ferociously stressed at this point! I hit the ramp and the vehicle aggressively accelerated to merge onto Route 18 going southbound, which is precisely the moment when it hit! The epileptic trigger held deep within started to surface warning my body that it was about to take on a seizure—only I hadn't a clue as to what the sophisticated sensation meant.

These epileptic episodes are extremely complex, often manifesting in different forms and sensations. The best way for me to explain the sensation in my case is that of déjà vu as the aura takes shape and grabs hold. Sometimes it ignites from a song that is stuck in my head, patterns of beats, sirens or emergency responders and fire/tornado whistles, a previous night's dream, seeing a color pattern, the feeling of excitement, or, in this case, the feeling of sheer stress. I know the feeling and onset all too well. At times it can be very light and almost euphoric as I bounce around the tingling sensation on my left side. It's sort of the feeling you get while smoking marijuana where you can bend and control the sensation. Sometimes the feeling is brutally strong, which causes a unique, dense odor in my nasal receptors. All sounds are amplified, and specific rhythm patterns are thick and exaggerated.

There are times when the intensity is so overpowering that a form of nausea occurs. The episodes typically last a few minutes but can be as short a few seconds, or I can feel the onset but then the feeling retreats akin to a sneeze that refuses to come to fruition. On occasion, several small bursts erupt rapidly, one after the other, for long periods of time. My Altoona high school graduation commencement comes to mind, when I had an intense aura throughout most of the ceremony, which was over an hour long. Powerful waves poured across my brain and into my body like crashing waves during high seas.

In the past, on occasion, I have operated a vehicle as the condition would set in. The onset typically passes within a few minutes, and that is that. So, as I merged in with the flow of traffic with my head full of activity, I turned the music down from the stereo and opened the windows just a crack to let some fresh air in. There was no time to slow down at a time like this and I knew the episode would pass in a few moments. "Just concentrate and stay focused," I thought to myself as I again picked up speed, briskly shifting to the passing lane. The feeling was pretty intense, and I knew that I simply had to compensate for a few more moments and surely the sensation would rush out of my body, the same as always. I hit the exit of the underpass, which was less bottled up than I had anticipated just minutes before. I exhaled a breath of relief. Now if I could just get through the blasted Commercial Avenue intersection, which was now only one mile away, I might pull off this miracle jaunt and arrive just a moment or so behind schedule.

I checked the time. It was minutes before noon. The throbbing brain waves were still consuming my senses to a degree. I could hear and feel the engine find the next gear; I heard the thick wind squeezing through the driver's side-window. I monitored the slight patterns of rhythm being generated from the faintly playing stereo. I looked up and noticed an incoming train pulling into the New Brunswick station from above, arriving from New York City, heading westbound. And then, a moment later, everything went pitch black.

5

WHERE IS MY MIND?

heard an indecipherable male voice coming from my right-hand side. My heavy eyes slowly opened and came back into focus. When I looked down, I was shocked! There was debris everywhere around me.

An image of a police officer's face came into my peripheral right. His lips were moving as if to communicate with me, but I couldn't make out his words. Everything was disorganized and chaotic. He must have been asking if I was all right, but I was unable to make any sense of it all. Was I all right? I simply didn't know.

Waves of sound began to flow and ebb. He instructed me not to move as he carefully opened the passenger door. I didn't move. Rather, I started to look around to get my bearings. The man speaking to me was a New Brunswick police officer. He said, "I'm going to help you get out of here, but you need to remain very still for a few minutes." I nodded my head, only semi-comprehending.

He reached through the passenger-side window and carefully opened the door. Now I saw that the debris was from the two blown-out airbags and that thick shards of glass lay all over me. The officer had smashed in the passenger-side window to get to me. "An ambulance will be here in a few minutes. Just stay calm. You're all right now."

I could hear and feel the chaos growing around. I heard the sirens in the distance, and then I looked out my rearview mirror. Traffic was at a standstill as far as the eye could see, and there now were multiple vehicles with flashing lights ahead of where I was positioned. I looked up and saw a traffic light changing from green to yellow to red as if nothing had happened on this brisk, yet sun-filled, February day.

Directly in front of me, about ten yards away and just through the intersection, there was an SUV stopped, and a woman was outside talking to another officer. To the left, I noticed that my rear driver's side was smashed up against a concrete barrier separating the southbound from the northbound lanes with the front jutting out past the concrete barriers into the intersection facing oncoming traffic.

The officer appeared again from the passenger side. He must have sensed that I was at least regaining my bearings when he calmly introduced himself and asked, "Where were you coming from?" In a state of confusion and uncertainty, I said, "Route 202." "Where were you going?" he naturally asked. I looked around dumbfounded and said, "Down the road for a meeting." Yet I had no memory as to exactly where I was going. The officer grabbed my cell phone, which was on the floor due to the impact. He instinctively hit the last call button and called the most recent number dialed, which of course was Mike Rodriguez from fifteen minutes earlier. Mike naturally picked up and the officer gave him specific instructions, which I wasn't following with all the pandemonium around me.

Within minutes, there was an entire first response fleet around me. Police cars, ambulances, and fire trucks parked off to the right-hand side of a construction zone. An EMT approached the smashed-out passenger side and asked me a series of questions. I offered little more than yes and no responses in my state of confusion. I looked up again at the traffic light and noticed the green sign in the center, which read "Commercial Avenue." I knew where I was! Then it hit me that the last thing I remembered was the train crossing the Raritan River above me before everything went dark.

The New Brunswick police and firefighters worked diligently to move my vehicle into the neutral gear in order to get me out. Several of these responders were leaning into my vehicle and giving me specific instructions not to move until otherwise instructed. My head and face were throbbing. Approximately ten minutes later, the officer returned to the passenger side-door. He leaned in and looked at me in an authoritative yet compassionate manner. "The EMTs are going to take good care of you from here. You'll be transported to Robert Wood Johnson Hospital, which is right around the corner. They'll get you checked out once you get over there. If you need anything, feel free to reach out. My name is Officer Ingram." He looked, over his left shoulder, for a moment at the wreckage behind then at the intersection in front of him. Then back at me, his expression tightening for a moment. "You don't know how lucky you were today, young man," he said, almost choking up it seemed. "We will check up with you later to see how you're doing."

I likely thanked him, but honestly, I have no recollection; nor did I remember his name. The goal now was to transfer me from my vehicle to the ambulance by way of a spinal board because they didn't know if I had injured my neck or spine. I tried to remain as still as possible while several responders worked assertively and briskly, as if they had this routine down to a science. My neck was put into a harness device; then they hoisted me out of the wreckage, strapping me to the board from my shoulders, chest, and legs. All of these safety measures were being conducted while in the middle of this extremely congested intersection. The sounds around me were very intense and overbearing. I was confused and overwhelmed. But most of all, I was frightened as to what had just happened. They gingerly transported me to the stretcher and then loaded me into the ambulance.

Once I was secured inside, the crew worked feverishly to stabilize me. As I recall, they somehow managed to remove my tie in one piece but had to use sheers to remove my dress shirt and undershirt to expose my chest as these suction cup devices were affixed above my heart, lungs, and abdomen. An oxygen tube was inserted into my nose and multiple IVs were stabbed into place to inject medicines and other solutions. One of the EMTs signaled up to the driver that all was in place and we were ready to go. I heard the sirens fire up and the ambulance pulled away from the crash site (which, to this day, I still refer to as my personal "Ground Zero"). I was completely overwhelmed as monitors blinked and beeped while other life support machines within the mobile unit sounded and signaled.

I believe that there were three people who hovered over me checking vitals. Each of them had a particular duty to perform, and everyone was amazingly calm. What I also remember vividly about the journey was that the very gentle woman who had applied my first IV started asking me a series of questions. How old are you? Are you married? Where do you work? What do you do for a living? Do you know what today's date is? What is your social security number? Who is the President of the United States? What time is it? And what is your address? I realized that many of these questions were just standard fact-finding protocol, but in the moment, I was unable to answer some of them. I forgot my address, my phone number, my social security number, who the president was, and even my wife's name. Sure, this was all extremely chaotic, but why couldn't I think correctly? I have an unparalleled long-term memory. What was happening in my head, goddammit? The woman told me to just relax and concentrate on my breathing. The entire ambulance ride took only five minutes. However, in that moment, it felt more like an eternity.

My sales rep Mike did exactly what Officer Ingram told him to do. He immediately called the office and told them that I was in some sort of auto accident on Route 18 southbound at Commercial

Avenue. He was also wise enough to relay the message that I was conscious and would be transported to nearby Robert Wood Johnson to get further evaluated.

When we hit the emergency room entrance, a fleet of medical professionals was awaiting our arrival. I felt the intensity heighten again. When the doors to the ambulance swung open, two doctors bolted into the back where I lay fastened to the stretcher. They immediately started asking the EMT crew questions about my condition, awareness, and medical history. I do recall specifically that the really nice lady told one of the doctors that I seemed to be a bit confused but in no way irrational or critical. The other doctor focused on my neck and spine, asking me if I could feel my fingers, toes, and jaw. I indeed could feel all three, I replied. A good sign, I thought, as they prepared my exit out of the ambulance. They put an absurdly bulky and heavy apparatus on a vacant area of my chest, which was not poked with electrodes and straps.

Upon entry into the hospital, the mood was still extremely tense. The staff whisked me past any sort of admissions check-in and straight back to an observation room where they immediately started swapping out IV bags, while switching the electrode cords that ran from my chest into a more advanced yet still portable type of machine. It immediately started beeping and flashing as the doctors were writing down notes and rigorously giving other instructions. My vitals were taken and to my knowledge checked out fine. Shortly after, they started analyzing my neck, asking me to raise my arms and wiggle my toes and so forth. All seemed to check out, and within twenty minutes or so the doctors ruled out that any sort of spinal cord injury had occurred. The assistants began to separate my body from the spinal board starting from my legs and demanding that if anything felt odd, to speak out immediately. Finally, the neck brace was removed. All was good on that front!

Now I was able to sit upright and was given one of those hospital smocks, so the doctors and nurses had easy access to my heart, lungs, back, and abdomen. I suppose at this point all checked out and they considered me to be in stable condition because everyone seemed to move on to other cases. It wasn't until another half hour or so when another doctor came into the room and began to look at the charts and forms. He was a nice younger guy and started to ask me a slew of questions as to how exactly I got here. By this point, I was thinking a bit clearer than I had been an hour ago. I regained memory of my phone number, date of birth, and simple current events. He asked me about my morning routine and if anything felt off. "Nope, just the typical day," I replied, trying to act nonchalant.

Author's Note:

I'm going to break off again right now and state a fact. I was not completely honest with this guy! I knew I'd had a spell in the car. Yet, in my defense, I had no way to describe the terminology for a neurological event of this nature. Also, how was I to know that the one event correlated with the other? I sort of figured that somehow this was all connected but, in that moment, I kept my mouth shut. This was not a smart move on my part!

★ ★ ★

By this time Christy, Doug, and Leon had arrived at the hospital and were permitted to see me. This put me in better spirits. It was also when the doctor, as well as my distinguished guests, started firing questions at me like a Civil War Gatling gun. Through the entire interrogation, I kept my little secret hidden. The doctor suggested that they run some tests because, obviously, I had lost consciousness at some point. What I did in fact tell them was that I remembered being fully alert until I went under the bridge where the trains ran. The doctor processed this statement for a moment. "So, what you are telling us is that you essentially drove almost a half mile completely unconscious?" "Yes," I responded. "Commercial Avenue is probably that distance from where it all went dark."

They all looked at one another dumbfounded. I thought that was a pretty impressive feat, despite the circumstances. "I am scheduling Jonathan for a CT scan immediately," the doctor stated in an authoritative tone. "Something is not adding up here". He grunted to himself while analyzing my blood test results. "How do you feel now?" the doctor asked me. "I feel fine, other than my head and the side of my face hurt. I'm still a little foggy and tired but fine nonetheless," I said. "I still want to run a CT scan" he insisted, and I agreed that was fine. Arrangements were made to have the scan done that evening. I was gaining an appetite throughout all of this waiting and pricking and checking and scheduling. Sandwiches were served until my number was called to head to the lab for scanning. I wasn't nervous in the least, just a bit achy and very tired. Naturally, I just wanted to get home after this long and strenuous day.

6

MASTER OF MY CRAFT

t all sounds like high-paced organized chaos, doesn't it? I get it. But I absolutely loved the pace! My job, my new wife of six months, my office, the culture of Worldwide Express, and my overall quality of life in the Garden State. I absolutely thrived in it all. There was a real buzz of opportunity as a twenty-eight-year-old entrepreneurial-minded, goal-driven sales professional. I liked the concept of building something big in a competitive environment (which in this case was a solid book of business, then a sales team).

The guys had promoted me to sales manager the year before, complete with a gifted BMW 530i and trip to Vegas (the shenanigans of those few days could likely be drafted into a memoir in itself). Our franchise numbers exploded from roughly $29,000 in weekly revenue sales into a two-and-a-half-year run of over $110,000 in weekly sales. We were crushing it in the Northeast, and the entire franchise system knew it! We worked hard; we played hard. My reps and I hit record growth numbers personally, and as an organization. That was mind blowing. We were recognized at our annual sales conferences year after year as we strutted onstage to pick up our awards and Happy Gilmore–sized checks while shaking the hands of the exec-level honchos and celebrities who emceed the evening. I was a workaholic. All I wanted to do was hang out with the gang at the office long after we called it a day. When Sunday hit, all I wanted to do was plan my Monday morning meetings.

When my reps and I would get thrown out of office buildings because of "No Soliciting" violations while cold calling, I used to bellow to the security guard or office manager who kicked us out or threatened us to leave, "Yeah? Yeah, Let's compare W-2s and see who sleeps better tonight." We'd then have a huge laugh once outside the quarters that we'd just gotten ejected from for the second time in two weeks. We would set up monthly sales contests that my team hit often, which typically consisted of stretch limousines, jet skis, exclusive golf courses, Kobe beef, seafood towers, and enough booze and fancy red wine to put down an adolescent gorilla.

We once had a conference in Scottsdale, Arizona, and the guys had the brilliant idea to celebrate in Vegas because we had hit our quarterly numbers a few months earlier. Hitting our projected numbers was always a big deal for our office, but this particular contest hit a revenue milestone. Doug, Leon, Greg, and I would already be out there anyway, so we made arrangements for Bobby, another tenured sales guy who stayed back, to fly into Vegas for the weekend. The four of us were going to drive the three hours from Arizona to Nevada, putting us at the Bellagio just in time to get the weekend burning.

Leon and Doug are truly "legit gamblers" in a casino environment. These are the guys who know the equations on how to work over the pit bosses into comping all sorts of high-end on-site dining establishments, and jazz on high-stakes tables. Not out-of-control stakes, mind you, but their speed is typically not sitting at $25.00 or $50.00 tables of blackjack where the waitresses stop by every ten minutes to see if they need a refreshment, if you catch my drift. These guys are full throttle. In my tenure with them, I've seen them win big and loose hard; yet, regardless of the outcome, they have no regrets and we always have a blast!

The larger and more elaborate operations out there have a system in place in which the casino acts essentially as a savings vehicle to their patrons so, in our case, the boys aren't flying and driving all over the country with 30k in cash. Leon, who at times has the attention span of a Cheerios box, was given the sole responsibility of ensuring that the funds would be properly wired and secured for distribution upon our arrival.

We checked in and then blasted into our respective rooms with excitement and anticipation of what these forty-eight hours would have in store. We were all located on the same floor and in very close proximity to one another. We arranged my room as the meet-up/pregame/postgame spot to easily account for everyone. As we got nestled in (nestled in meaning ravaging the contents of each rooms minibar), the guys came in from their quarters directly across the hall and told us that they were heading down to retrieve the capital and we should stay in place and wait for Bobby to arrive within the hour. A half hour or so went by as we marveled over the epic Bellagio fountains, Caesars Palace, and other grand landmarks looking up and down the Las Vegas Strip. Victory toasts were given; tiny bottles of spiced rum along with canned beers were distributed evenly. It was the perfect little gathering before the party officially hit high gear. And then at some point in the hype of the pre-celebration, my phone rang. . . .

It was Doug. He sounded concerned. "What's up?" I said. "Jonathan, is Leon at your room yet?" He wasn't. "Jonathan, if he gets there before me, do not let him out of that room!" OK, but why? "Because if he comes back down here, we're all probably going to get kicked out of the hotel."

I noticed a silence come over the room. "When he gets here, I won't let him leave," I vowed, then hung up and simply said that

Doug was acting frantic about something and he would be up shortly. A few minutes passed. Suddenly, Leon practically kicked the door down (we had all the doors partially ajar for our crew coming in and out), heading straight for the minibar. "These fuckers are all full of shit!" he snarled as he pulled out two small bottles of Johnny Walker Red and gulped them down aggressively.

"Doug just called and said that you're supposed to stay here," I instructed, trying my best to be authoritative. "What the hell is going on?"

He just stood there, spitting nails while pounding his double scotch. Something about how the front desk had screwed up. I started to put the pieces together. Doug got to the room a few minutes later. He was pissed, and Leon wouldn't even look at him. "So, what are we supposed to do now?" Doug questioned. "I don't know. Have those stunads at the desk figure it out!" Leon roared.

"What's going on?" again I asked. Apparently, Leon did not take all the steps necessary to complete the wire transfer of the funds. To make matters worse, it was Friday evening in Vegas, which was far past the bank's closing time to clear up the matter. Even worse than that was that Leon and Doug were smart enough to never take personal credit cards to these types of establishments. Bottom line, we were stuck in Las Vegas with little more than a few American Express Platinum Cards to get us through this debacle. "Let's pull funds from our AMEXs," I suggested. "You cannot pull cash advances via cards through American Express," Doug educated me, which is the very reason why Doug and Leon always traveled with nothing other than that particular card. Doug, who is always the voice of reason, suggested that we all go down to the sports book and grab some drinks so we could pull ourselves together and wait for Bobby to arrive. So that's what we did.

Leon finally "sort of" admitted that he'd screwed up leaving us in the predicament that we were in. We were just going to have to make the best of it. We all calmed down and started to reminisce about how we had gotten here in the first place. Bobby had gotten into town by this point and we were contemplating dinner plans while telling tales of hilarity in a now booze-fueled state. At one point, a conversation about credit card debt and finances was pointed my way. I have always been very strict and disciplined when it comes to credit card debt. Doug and I have talked about finances of this nature and he has been a great mentor on that front. A moment later, he asked me about a conversation we'd had a week prior regarding how he wanted me to barter with one of the credit card companies to extend balance limits, reduce the interest rate, and increase the line of credit, and asked me if I had followed through with it. "Well, of course I did," I said. "So, you have a line of credit on that card, correct?" "Yes, I do." Out of the corner of my eye I could see Leon's wheels churning. "You have that card on you currently, don't you?" Now I could see where this was going, fast!

In old movies you sometimes see the gold phones gleaming in gambling establishments. Well, I'm here to tell you that those phones really do exist (typically around the corner from the cashier booth). When it was all through, I had taken out a twenty-one-thousand-dollar cash advance! I pleaded with Leon that my wife was going to kill me when she found out about this. He told me not to worry and he would take care of the situation as soon as we got back to the office on Monday. Sure enough, the weekend went on in grandiose style. Funds were won and burned on that trip and we all had a blast. And, sure enough, a check of reimbursement and then some was put in my hands on the following day of business at the office.

Were girlfriends, fiancées, and wives becoming irritated at times with our shenanigans? Sure they were! It doesn't exactly set the mood when you arrive back home at two thirty in the morning via the local cab service and come crawling into bed smelling of lobster butter and bourbon, I tell you. Benders of this proportion were not all that frequent, truth be told. But we celebrated wins both big and small back then in the New Jersey Central office. It was all harmless fun that glistened a small stone of youthful success and loyalty to the duo that took the entrepreneurial plunge very early into their professional careers. These were some of the greatest, comical, and most outrageous experiences of my life to date (and as you can only imagine, I've done some pretty wild shit!). Simply reflecting on the plethora of tales can spin my stomach into half-hour-long laughing fits to this day.

7

I DREAM OF JESUS

The nurse came to fetch me for my CT scan at a little past 8:00 P.M. I was taken via wheelchair (which I thought was completely unnecessary but supposed it was protocol) and was debriefed as to the purpose of the scan. The procedure was explained to be a routine, relatively quick and painless process, which combines several X-rays to produce a detailed image of structures inside the body. The results would be obtained within a half hour and then be translated by a doctor.

The entire process front to back took no longer than twenty minutes. I was wheeled back to the observation area, from which I had been originally parked nine hours earlier. Christy was still there, making necessary phone calls and arrangements. She instructed Doug and Leon to go home and that she would update them as information was released. By this point, I was brutally exhausted, and the side of my face now began to show signs of swelling.

Finally, at around nine o'clock, a different doctor came back and began to ask a lot of the same questions that had been asked hours before. My accounts of the day's events were consistent with the earlier testimony. He told me to hold tight (as if there was anything else for me to do) and we would figure out a game plan from here. Well, this seemed to be a bit confusing for Christy and me. We were just assuming that all would check out and this would be written off as a fluke incident of sorts. After ten minutes, the doctor came in with another doctor and started to talk about the results of the scan.

The second doctor was a neurologist, which is a doctor who specializes in the functionality of the nervous system. The two professionals started to riff off one another as if to almost validate each of their respective accreditations in front of us while explaining their findings. After a few minutes of technical doctor jargon, they finally started to get to the point. "What your scan results are showing is that there seems to be some type of growth around the front temporal lobe of your brain." "We cannot confirm or speculate on the nature of it without additional testing. This is not always a bad prognosis; rather, we simply do not know as of yet." So that was that. Or so I thought.

"I want to keep him overnight and perform an MRI scan in the morning to get a better understanding as to what is going on in there," said the neurologist. The difference between a CT scan and an MRI is that an MRI uses powerful magnetic fields and radio frequency pulses to produce detailed pictures of organs, soft tissue, bones, and internal body structures. So an MRI is often cleaner than a CT scan.

My first thought, naturally, was, "Son of a bitch! What do you mean that you're keeping me in the pen for the night?"

Here's what I said: "How about this for a game plan? You folks let me go home, I'll get a good night's rest, I'll take this ice pack home to reduce the swelling on my face, and we will meet you back here tomorrow morning for you to run all the tests that you desire?" "No can do, sir," number two white coat said. "We need that IV line in place to inject a dye for the testing tomorrow. Just a night to see what is going on up there," he persisted. "And I hear they serve a great breakfast in the morning," he said in a jovial fashion.

"You bastard," I surely thought.

Arrangements were made, bands with general information were fastened to my right wrist, and I was an official resident of Robert Wood Johnson Hospital for the evening. Honestly, I was so exhausted from the day's events that all of this didn't really matter. I sent Christy home and demanded that she not make a big deal out of this little incident to mothers or siblings back in Pennsylvania.

* * *

I had to hand it to the guy. He was correct about the breakfast spread in this joint! I woke up well rested at 8:30 A.M. to nurses checking vitals while they made me scarf down a made-to-order omelet, home fries, toast, orange juice, muffins, and fruit. Christy showed up shortly after and so began my Saturday. My body was sore all over from the vehicle accident the day prior. The pain medication given the night before had apparently worn off because the left side of my face hurt something awful. Now all there was to do was sit and wait for the MRI to be executed. The plan would go as follows: Get all this preventative testing over with, understand the results given, comply with all instructions and preventative measures recommended, give my personal gratitude to all who were involved over the past twenty-four-hour debauchery, and enjoy what was left of the weekend while getting ready for what would be a very busy Monday morning at the office. It wasn't until close to noon when they informed the nurses that I was scheduled for the test. I was ready with bells on when the guy showed up. He brought a wheelchair into the room and asked my name. I jumped up and hunkered in to be whisked down halls and elevators, then more halls, all the while making small talk with my personal chauffer until we got to a congested waiting area that was four beds deep with patients of all ages. He told me that an assistant would take me from here and they would call for him to retrieve me once the testing was over. "Fair enough," I said, and patiently waited my turn in line, which ended up taking well over an hour to get me into the prep area. I was then instructed to remove my watch and wedding band before heading into a room with a large circular machine and a toboggan-looking table on which the technician prompted me to lie down faceup and put a mask-type contraption (which I could see out of) over my face. Finally, they gave me a device to hold and squeeze if I needed assistance or felt uncomfortable. The toboggan table then began to slide backward, placing me inside the tube about up to my waist. The technician, now in a separate room where she could conduct the scan through a glass partition, told me to lie still.

For the most part, I was comfortable in the tube. I dozed off at times and never felt claustrophobic. It all sounded like a bunch of clicking and banging as the machine moved to precise coordinates on my head. I simply lay there motionless for the required twenty minutes as the contraption collected the necessary data. Minutes after the scan was over, the same buddy who'd brought me down came to wheel me back up to my room to await my results.

When we got back to my room, I had a most unexpected visitor awaiting my return. My sense of sight and sound came together to recognize the voice that was chatting with Christy as the nurses transferred me back into bed. "Do you remember me?" he asked. His uniform sort of gave away his disguise though. "I remember you from yesterday," I said. It was none other than Officer Ingram, who had fulfilled his promise of checking in on me. "They made a couple calls yesterday and one again this morning informing us that you were still admitted so I thought I'd drop by for a few minutes and see how you're holding up," he said. "I didn't expect to be here this long," I said, rolling my eyes to the back of my head. "It's all protocol, I suppose."

"I'm sure they'll get you buttoned up in no time," he assured me. Officer Ingram slid around the bottom of the bed to get a closer view of me. He then sat on the chair beside my bed as we started to make light conversation for a few minutes. Then he changed the subject. I could tell that something was on his mind. He asked me to recount yesterday's events both before I lost consciousness and after I woke up at the intersection. I immediately asked if I was in trouble for something. "No, No, not in the least," he affirmed. "I did tell you how lucky you were that the accident wasn't far worse." Yes, he had. "Do you remember any parts between going blank and coming to?" he continued. "Not anything," I said. He shifted in his chair. "Do you remember the blue SUV that went through the intersection ahead of you?" "Yes, yes, I do!" I was excited about this because I truly did remember. "There was a woman talking to another officer beside a blue SUV!" "Yes," he affirmed. He took a deep breath and then exhaled. "That vehicle and the woman driving it are the reason why your accident wasn't far worse," he said, his eyes firmly on me. "Oh?" I said, not being able to really process what he was implying. "That could have been tragic." He began to relay the woman's account of the events.

At approximately the time that I had fallen unconscious, my vehicle was using the passing lane when, moments later and for no apparent reason, the vehicle jolted. The front left of my vehicle slammed off of the concrete slab running down the center of the highway. The traffic behind began to slow drastically, but the vehicle was apparently maintaining speed upwards of 50 mph. The woman sped up to get out ahead of the "so-called erratic driving behavior," but when she passed, she noticed that my head was unconsciously beating off of the driver's-side window. My hands were on the wheel, but obviously something was seriously wrong as the front end smacked off of the concrete again and again, now with smoke and mist spewing out of the engine block and a path of debris beginning to build with no sign of deceleration or braking. The highway curvature graded left, which in a current trajectory would not provide much of a barrier to slow the now-out-of-control missile on wheels. The SUV braked once more to confirm what she had assumed (now she noticed that the airbags were deployed), then she propelled to a safe distance in front of the tattered vehicle. From her driver's-side mirror, she could hear and see that even though the speed was declining, the engine was revving at high levels, meaning my foot was still applied to the gas even as the vehicle was beating against the barrier. She immediately took action. Assuming at this point the vehicle had decelerated to somewhere between twenty to thirty miles per hour thirty seconds into this episode, something had to be done. She aligned the SUV right rear bumper with the left front of my vehicle. The bumpers struck and she hit the brakes, pinning me against the concrete barrier and her vehicle. Moments later, both automobiles came screeching to a halt. We were positioned a mere three feet before the barrier ended at the intersection of Commercial Avenue.

I was flabbergasted by the officer's words. The events of the day prior could have been filled with far more dire consequences. Officer Ingram could hardly believe the words that he was speaking himself. I could tell he was having trouble processing it all. "You definitely had an angel looking down on you yesterday, my friend." I felt a shiver go through my body as my eyes became noticeably heavy. At that moment, I realized what tragedy was prevented by an act of impromptu thinking and bravery. I immediately asked if he could get us her information so that I could contact her. Officer Ingram shifted his posture once more. "She gave us her information because with any matter of this nature a report must be drafted, but she did give my fellow officer specific instructions that this matter was over, and she asked not to be contacted regarding this incident."

I was dumfounded by this. "Well, I need to contact her!" I demanded. He rose from the chair knowing that his words would tear through me and settle forever. He rose and turned away. "Some people simply don't want to be bothered," he said earnestly.

A few more formalities were addressed between the three of us. I thanked him for all he did for me and he told me to reach out to him directly if I needed anything further.

Author's Note:

We retrieved the official police report completed by Officer Ingram from the afternoon of the accident. The contact name of the woman involved was included. Multiple attempts were made in the following days, weeks, and months to reach out and shower her with words of appreciation and gratitude for her loving act of bravery and kindness. None of our messages were ever returned. In my opinion, this unlikely heroine was given a situation and handled it to the best of her ability. That was all. I think about her all the time. God holds a special place for her in heaven. I am quite sure of this.

★ ★ ★

A few hours later, we were informed that my MRI results from the lab were complete and a doctor would be in shortly to discuss. After the visit with Officer Ingram, I practically forgot about the scan that had been done that morning. It was getting later in the afternoon and I had to order lunch from downstairs. I had in the back of my head already that each meal ordered translated to several more hours before they discharged me. It was almost Saturday evening by this point and I was jonesing to get the results and get the hell out of this place at a decent hour.

Soon, yet another doctor gingerly knocked a few times on the door and entered the room carrying a whole slew of binders and documents. He was an older gentleman who was very blunt and to the point. He did not have any form of bedside manner and walked in as if he were going to give a PowerPoint presentation to an audience. Every other professional to this point had been incredible as far as giving us updates and all in all just making me feel as comfortable as possible until we could get this ordeal over with. This Dr. Berman character was about as exciting as a post hole digger. "Regardless, get the lecture underway and get me outta here!" was all I could think about as he began to position large X-ray-looking images on a lighted examination board that was affixed to the wall beside my bed.

He announced his presence and credentialed himself as a neurosurgeon associated with the hospital. He began to explain all the intricacies as to how the MRI results are presented and how a professional who specializes in neurological conditions interprets the data shown. "OK, buddy, let's get on with it!" I fidgeted around impatiently as he started to explain the first image on the screen.

The images were insanely graphic views of my brain. They were so granular that one could see the eye sockets and nasal orifice from multiple views and angles. It is truly amazing to view your cranium from the top down on the inside. Once he got done explaining the medical jargon of the scan, he pointed to the front right section of the skull using his pen as a pointer. "You will notice this black mass on the right, just above the eye socket, which is called the front temporal lobe. Not only should it not be there, but also it could be causing pressure to build up against the skull. This is likely a cyst that caused the tonic-clonic episode otherwise known as grand mal seizure." He turned to us, speaking authoritatively.

That's about all that needed to be said. This was so much more serious than I had first thought. Was this the demon that was causing the brain activity that I had experienced all those years? My brain raced into overdrive, thinking about all sorts of theories and assumptions. Even so, I still would not speak about the episode that had caused the blackout igniting the accident. "There simply must be a correlation between the brain activity and the accident," I thought. "There is no other rational explanation!"

I realized at this point that I would not be receiving the "You're in good shape, young man! You are free and clear to leave this evening." This was very, very serious.

"So, what are we going to do here, Doc?" I asked in a half jovial, half scared shitless manner. "I am going to present the results to a small panel of fellow neurologists early next week," he replied. "There seems to be pressure on the wall of the brain caused by a cyst of some nature, which is likely the result of the epileptic event that you endured." "Well, what the hell does that mean?" I thought. "If indisputable evidence is agreed upon, we will operate as soon as all testing checks out, which likely will be early next week." He nodded in affirmation and then left.

Author's Note:

This marks the beginning of the slew of medical terminology that I realized was pertinent to absorb and understand. As we all know by this point, I am far from an "attention to detail" personality. Rather, I have a fly-by-the-seat-of-my-pants, it-will-work-itself-out-when-needed mindset, which doesn't work well when dealing with this sort of subject matter. I was fortunate to have Christy there as she instinctively grabbed a notepad and pen and started rigorously writing down pertinent points of the discussion. The more eyes and ears that you have in these types of settings, the better. If I were in that room by myself, I would not have understood two-thirds of the medical terminology that was thrown at me (mainly because I was afraid to ask). Furthermore, if I had to pass on the information effectively at a later point, let's just say that it would have been a disaster.

The two terms that flashed through my head as the doctor concluded his findings were *frontal lobe* (the front of the brain) and *cyst* (fluid-filled sac). This was rhetoric that I had heard years before.

* * *

That evening, the warning rockets were fired. Christy sent news to our families, and friends back home were informed of the news that somehow spread like wildfire through central Pennsylvania. Doug and Leon were obviously debriefed as well. I wasn't all that concerned about the news, to be honest, once Berman left and I had some time to digest it all. From what I interpreted, he didn't seem all that concerned either. Sure, this was a serious matter, but he didn't seem to flinch as he explained the situation to us. After all, he made a point that he was very familiar with this sort procedure; he had performed it many times.

This entire twenty-four-hour ordeal was starting to get to me by this point. First of all, I learned rather quickly that hospitals run skeleton crew shifts on weekends (which makes sense). And now they were keeping me admitted through the beginning of next week to be monitored. The whole state of affairs was turning out to be fucking brutal! "These bastards are not going to make me miss work on Monday," I scowled. I was hot! Yet, I knew that I wasn't getting out of here without some sort of massive correctional action being performed. I wanted two items at that moment—my journal and at least one of my acoustic guitars. The journal was doable and would at least help me pass some time. Christy went home and returned with sets of relaxation attire and writing materials to keep me entertained. She would stay with me for as long as visiting hours permitted and then some, and I would turn in at the ungodly hour of 9:00 P.M. only to be routinely woken up for vital checks by nurses at 11:00 P.M., 2:00 A.M., 5:00 A.M., and 8:00 A.M.

I found sleep to be surprisingly difficult those first couple of nights. There seemed to be a constant wave of noise pollution from the hallways and nurses' station that you couldn't seem to block out fully no matter if the door was open or shut. Machines, and call buttons, and the sounds of emergency vehicles pulling up to the building, and people moaning and crying. One positive that I forgot to mention is that they were nice enough to give me a room to myself, making me wonder as I look back why I couldn't have my guitar up there to riff around on at a reasonable hospital-acceptable noise level!

The left side of my face bruised up something impressive over the next two days. The only thing that looked more impressive was the track marks that were forming on both arms from multiple IV puncture wounds and needle piercings from what felt like quarts of blood being extracted for testing purposes. Besides another CT scan on Sunday morning, the daily routine began to set in at this point. The one positive in all this was that I had no restrictions in terms of being confined to either my bed or room, so roaming the halls and writing in common areas filled up painfully slow-moving days. I would eat three solid meals per day because the food was still quite palatable. My mom, sister Katie, mother-in-law, and sister-in-law had arrived the evening prior, and fellow comrades from the office would stop by to kill a couple hours at a time as well.

An awesome part of those days that comes to mind was waking up from a nap to find a whole slew of the Bellmeade Drive crew in my room. Someone made the arrangements with Christy the day before and a handful of them made the six-hour jaunt to cheer up a beat-up soldier in a time of need. I was so pumped to see those clowns! We laughed and told ridiculous tales of our youth as we burned up the afternoon in a common area downstairs. When it was time for them to go, I got a bit bummed out because it was back upstairs to the same ol' same ol'. It was an incredible gesture on their part and just another example of how tight that crew from back home remains to this day. My office team was great as well! They knew this whole experience was hitting me hard. The news that I would not be returning for a few days made it that much worse and they knew it.

Finally, on Monday morning, things were back to normal here at "the rock." The full staff was back, and by this point I knew faces and names of many on my floor. Now, yet again, we were in a holding pattern waiting anxiously for Dr. Berman to return with his counsel's debriefing, which happened at around eight that evening. My family assembled in my room and he began the consultation with where he had left off. His tone was stern and rigorous as he affirmed his findings from Friday. "I met with my associates this afternoon and we have unanimously agreed that the cyst should be extracted and biopsied to prevent further pressure from building around the mass. Furthermore, we will be able to retrieve tissue samples to determine if the mass shows any form of malignant [cancerous] properties." Immediately and deliberately, I looked at my mother, and our eyes locked when he made this statement. We both knew what the other was thinking. This was not the part of the debriefing that either of us wanted to hear—a result of events from five years earlier. This was the moment when my stomach tightened with knots while my left leg shook slightly with signs of nervous tension. It was so much to take in at that moment. "I cannot make my mom and sisters go through this." The tension in that small room was incredibly thick as we all looked at one another's faces and silently tried to gauge each other's emotional states as if playing a serious hand of poker. I spoke first in an attempt to execute the eight-hundred-pound gorilla in the room. I looked back at my mom, then Christy, and finally at Berman, nodded, and said authoritatively, "If this is what has to be done, let's go in and get it out!"

I don't recall much of the next thirty minutes of Q and A and timelines, which were explained in detail while I sat on the chair across from my bed and took the moment in. Everyone had a chance to put their two cents in and Berman would answer all questions accordingly. Nurses began to enter the room with documentation to be filled out and signed off on. The one part I did particularly pay attention to was when someone asked, "What are the potential side effects?" Despite all of the commotion going on in the room, I did stop to listen to what the doctor had to say. "Again, this procedure is quite common to my area of expertise. Typically, there are no side effects from this procedure other than some potential weakness on the left-hand side and soreness due to any type of invasive surgery such as this. "When can I go back to work?" was all that was on my mind. "If everything goes according to plan, you should be back to a normal lifestyle in two weeks or shortly thereafter. We need to remove the front right portion of the skull in order to uncover the cyst. It will take a period of time for the bones of the skull to fuse and realign so any sort of aggressive extracurricular activities are strictly prohibited!" Berman said. I forced myself to have a clear mindset at this point. "Fuck it! If I can put all of this behind me and be back to the office in a week and a half, let's do this!" All of these decisions were molded into a plan of action very rapidly. Getting a second opinion was never really considered. Looking back, if I would have spoken up about the aura activity that I had tolerated for most of my life, perhaps those conversations would have been different.

It was agreed upon that the surgery would be performed on Wednesday morning. I thought, "I'll be all sore, tired, and medicated up to my eyeballs anyway, so I won't even notice. Then it will be time to leave and I can at least recuperate within the confines of my own home." The masterfully developed plan was beginning to take shape nicely! A surgery-prepping exercise would be administered on Tuesday evening to line up electrodes on my skull with graphing technology on their end to make sure my skull was aligned precisely where the incision was to be created.

By the time the consultation was adjourned, it was getting late. Everyone's face seemed to be glazed over from information overload. The sheer exhaustion of the last couple of hours was starting to set in. It was my job to reassure my family that what we had decided was indeed the best decision (and I knew in the back of my head that this wasn't going to get any better). I was tired myself at this point and just wanted a bit of alone time to take everything in. We said our goodbyes and I journaled. From what I remember, I slept well that evening minus all of the blood pressure checking, beeping, blood drawing, and temperature taking on me and all around me.

* * *

If one was to think that day five was any more interesting than the prior four had been on the fourth floor of Robert Wood Johnson, you'd be fooling yourself.

Between waves of friends, family, and colleagues dropping by periodically all day, I still made my rounds saying hello and making small talk with the familiar faces on the ward—only today I had a slight burst of extra energy telling my fellow mates and professionals that even though I was going under the knife tomorrow morning, I'd be outta here soon thereafter. And everyone was happy for me. Most everyone who was involved by this point stopped by or called to wish me the best and a speedy recovery and all that jazz.

At around 7:00 P.M., they took me downstairs for the operation preparation exercise, which consisted of profiling the right side of my head on a table monitor where a visual grid appeared. The two technicians skillfully positioned between eight to twelve quarter-sized foam medallions (which reminded me of those white Life Saver mints) at random positions starting above my right eye and extending back behind my right ear. They explained that, tomorrow morning, the technicians would shave this entire area and the foam medallions would be reapplied showing Berman exactly where to break through to retrieve the mass. Once this prep was finished, I was whisked away and brought back upstairs. We arrived in my room to find yet another pack of well-wishers. To my delight, there was a fantastic spread of food that had arrived from the local restaurant, which we frequented often and which was conveniently located beside our complex. Our buddy Harold, the head chef, had caught wind of the next day's events and brilliantly coordinated a feast in my honor to make sure I had a good meal before my beheading come dusk! I laughed, thinking about him and his act of kindness. The mood was light. I boasted to all that were in shouting distance that this was officially "my last supper," and naturally no one knew how to react to that. Regardless, we ate and laughed and carried on even though I could detect the concern and uneasiness in the room. A nurse showed up at some point in the midst of festivities to inform us that a tech would be coming to fetch me by seven in the morning for prep, then surgery, so no more to eat now and plenty of rest until then.

Eventually, everyone said their goodbyes and all was quiet as this pre-surgery night set in. I wrote a little because, somehow, I knew that this would settle me in and calm me. When I dug it up these years later, I was pleased to find it was an entry that was short and to the point. I'd had enough of this environment. Whatever was in my head was not meant to be there and it needed to be removed. I needed to get back to my wife and my work. I had missed my guitars something awful over these past five days.

Journal Entry: February 20, 2006

What is deserved is an explanation of sorts: Where this deal began. I remember vividly being probably 5 years old standing on the other side of my parents' bed (ugly rose bedspread) the first time it happened. It is only defined as what one would call a slight déjà vu with an inner body pulsing reaction. The brain processes internal motions to external sequences. It has always seemed to be a random, unexpected event that comes and passes from time to time. The big one I got was at High school graduation that lasted at least a half hour. I had one at Jerk's (Bellmeade) driveway while playing basketball that evening after school. A most recent intense surge came over me at the Applegate Farms appointment with Mike Rodriguez. Who the hell comes up to say it is a medical diagnosis? I have told one person about the spells—that being Puddin' (yet another degenerate Bellmeade Drive Character, whose artistic wizardry actually created the cover art for this project). I mentioned the spells that my head fell into from time to time as we drove back home from the small town of Patten, Pa. late in the evening interpreting the lyrics to "Remembering the Mountain Bed." It's to be implied that I had a strong attack earlier this evening. I felt the need that I needed to tell someone just in case something went drastically wrong with me from within.

Journal Entry: February 21, 2006

So tomorrow they're going in. At this moment I'm a little on edge. All in all, I'm just ready to get this over with. Dr. Berman has got me covered and the staff here is great! I'm just sick of the sick. Goddamn pints of blood and IVs and blood pressure. It makes you want to just go back to work. This morning I woke up to The Bellmeade Crew at the foot of my bed. That was yet another one of the nicest things that anyone has ever done for me. We are a tight unit. Most do not understand that. The guys from the office came in after work and we had our Tuesday meeting. Doug and Leon have been by every day. Leon especially (as expected) has been stopping in regularly, which means the world to me. Mom, Rosie, Katie, and Gretchen came along for the ride as well. So here is the deal, most don't realize how long I have dealt with this and it is time to end. I know that the doctors and God will take care of me. I simply ask for a smooth operation. And shit, you've gotta think, the absolute worst-case scenario is that Dad, Uncle Frank, and I will be hanging out by 3:30 tomorrow afternoon. And how bad would that be?

On the morning of surgery, I was awake and ready for the day's festivities before the nurses came into my room to awaken me around five thirty. My family arrived within the hour as well. The mood was light and I was in fine spirits for the most part. Yeah, maybe a little nervous as the time drew near. "Let's just get this finished!" was the slogan that rang through my head that morning.

Prep technicians were now in the room doing their jobs while the nursing staff assisted. They all treated me as if I were the in-flight commander from an Apollo mission, I thought while they took my vitals and hooked up me up with yet another IV in my right arm. The room began to grow tense—perhaps far more tense than what I had anticipated. I again said what I could to calm everyone down while trying to keep the mood light with banter. Then a different nurse entered the room. She was precise in her words as she outlined what the day would look like. "When we take Jonathan downstairs for anesthesia and final prep, family members may come down until the anesthetist is ready for him. The duration of the operation will depend on several factors, but a nurse will keep everyone updated once information becomes available. Jonathan will then be taken to a recovery area while the anesthesia wears off. Dr. Berman and his staff can closely monitor his progress post-procedure. Once cleared within a couple hours, Jonathan will be taken to the ICU unit where he will likely stay for one to two nights until his condition is upgraded. Once he's given noncritical status, he shall return to the fourth floor to await further screening. Then final discharge recommendations will be carried out upon Dr. Berman's approval. Speaking of the doctor, you should plan for him to drop by Jonathan's room in the ICU tomorrow afternoon or evening, if I were to guess, to give further updates as well as biopsy results of the mass that is extracted."

I told her that sounded great. She continued, "I'm going to give the go-ahead for anesthesia on your say-so and we will be back to take you down to the operating level very soon." I nodded and gave her a thumbs-up. The woman left the room, and that was that. Then the nurses suited me up in yet another one of those ridiculous gowns, and within minutes, a different employee came to collect me on a very sophisticated bed with rollers, which was far different than the typical rolling beds I was used to. This one had several bells and whistles, and I was informed that this device reclined into a table from which they would conduct the operation. I hurled myself on to the contraption and my family began to file out of the room, heading for the elevators.

The guy who transported me down was a great fella, as I remember. He kept the mood light as I was likely making ridiculous banter. He played along with my wit as we made our way through the labyrinth of endless hallways and elevators.

Once on the operating floor, he wheeled me down a series of hallways until we came to a small holding area similar to where the MRI and CTI scans were performed. Only this time, my bed was the only one in the waiting area. He gave me a thumbs-up and I shot him two back. A few moments later, a relatively young guy in scrubs walked out of the two automatic swinging doors that were directly in front of me. He checked my wristband, making sure that the person in front of him was indeed the intended patient, and then introduced himself as my anesthetist. He said it would take him about five minutes to prepare the room and then we would be on our way.

"Great, glad to be here!" I said, attempting yet again to calm a nervousness from those around me that was so thick it was now making me uneasy. He walked back behind the doors. So now, as you can imagine, with some of the most important women in my life around me, I saw the tears begin to flow and heard the melancholy sobs from what I thought was to be my uplifting cheerleading squad! I saw my sister-in-law, Gretchen, first. She looked as if she had just witnessed a bulldozer accidently running over a litter of newborn kittens. She was an absolute mess! As I went down the line of loving women in my life, I reassured each that this was going to turn out just fine. "This is simply not going to be that big of a deal!" I reminded them as well as myself between hugs and an abundance of kisses that were applied to my forehead.

After the others said their "We'll see you in a few hours," Christy approached the side of my bed. I extended my left hand and placed her right hand in mine. I didn't need to say much. She was fighting back tears. "You know I'll be fine," I said. "I know you will," she affirmed as the words choked her. She then took my wedding band off, which made me ponder the absurdity of these circumstances a mere six months after our nuptials had been carried out. It all felt like a ridiculous joke being played on us by something that was far out of our control. She kissed me and held my hand as, just a moment later, my buddy came out and announced that I was all his from here. I began to hear the sniffles and the whimpers crescendo as he got behind my bed and started to push me toward the automatic doors, which flung open on his command. I likely made some sort of asinine yet warm-natured parting comment to my small entourage as he picked up the necessary momentum to maneuver me through the entryway. I heard every emotion in those final moments. Their presence began to fade once I was in the prep room. I thought about each one of them individually. And then, just like that, I heard the automatic doors collapse shut.

The prep room was a buzzing area of lights, sounds, and surgeon types each done up in scrubs and sophisticated masks. It was very bright. My anesthetist had his back to me as we were engaged in some form of simple-minded conversation. "How are you holding up?" he asked. "Did you see the looks of those women out there? I'm ready to get this over with." I responded sarcastically. "Are you going to knock me out?" I inquired. "Yes, I am, and the anesthesiologist will be close by just in case the surgeon needs him," he reassured me. "Did you sleep well last night amongst all this?" he inquired. "Not bad," I replied. "Well, in a few minutes, I'm going to pump you with a concoction that has a street value of around five grand that will knock you out cold!" I looked at him, perplexed. "If that's the case, what the hell are we doing here? Let's get down to Trenton and hawk this shit!" He howled with laughter and seemed to appreciate my upbeat attitude at this tough moment. He began to connect IV lines to bags of solution that were hanging above the bed. "All right, buddy," he soothed me. "The doc's team will be in to get you shortly. Are you ready?" he asked. "I am," I said. He prepared the shot and said, "When I inject this, I want you to take slow, deep breaths. You'll feel tired within a few moments, and before you know it, this will all be over." "Sounds good to me." I smiled and nodded. He pierced the skin with the solution and then rapidly connected the IV line on my left-hand side. I was marveling at his work while monitoring my breathing, just as he'd told me. And suddenly, it all went dark and I was under.

8

WONDERFUL

B efore we get too far ahead of ourselves, allow me to back up a bit. Summers on Bellmeade Drive were like no other. Our parents had an extremely lax approach when it came to rules such as checking in and curfew. Sleeping in, gathering at a specific time and place to play sports, having adventures in the woods, carrying out minor acts of mischief, and soaking up entire afternoons in someone's backyard swimming pool were all in the formula back then. The tether extended even more once we had our own transportation in the form of bicycles. At times we would tell the truth to our mothers as far as the day's itinerary, and at times we'd flat out lie with a destination or rally point being some eight miles across town for a game of pickup basketball or hanging out with friends or girls or girlfriends when puberty miraculously set in. The only rules were that there was no swimming permitted before baseball games (which was put into place by our coaches and fathers, yet held just about as much clout as our mothers' enforcing that we make sure to wait thirty minutes before jumping back into the pool after you eat or we'll surely drown sorta absurdity) and that you had to get home for dinner, which I typically abided by. There was always something to do and always a crew to carry on with. There were pockets of male adolescent youth all over that road. If I got bored, I'd simply get on my bike and ride around for a bit. Something always was happening somewhere. We were all into sports in some capacity as well, which kept us roped in most of the time anyway.

Some of our group were exceptionally talented, both athletically and academically, and some were not. I fell into the latter half of that camp. It was around age ten that I started to develop an extreme appreciation of music. Boom boxes, break dancing, DJ Jazzy Jeff and the Fresh Prince, and the Beastie Boys were the craze. I found the freedom of expression paired with musical talent to be invigorating back then. A couple years later, when MTV was added to standard cable packages due to popular demand all over the world, the hook was set instantly with me. I liked most music genres when I was young, but hard rock really grabbed me once I entered my teenage years. The whole "Parents Music Resource Center" founded by Tipper Gore was still in full swing so you needed to be sly when watching the legit music television videos or purchasing cassettes that were on the PMRC list. Nevertheless, I would stealthily watch late-night MTV programs such as Riki Rachtman's *Headbangers Ball* or Matt Pinfield's *120 Minutes* in the privacy of my bedroom basement. My parents were completely oblivious to the "musical acid rock" that I was mainlining into my brain for several hours on any given day. But listen, damnit, I want my MTV! The music scenes from coast to coast were fascinating to me. The overdriven guitars, intensity and volume of certain lead singers, power of a bass drum and crash cymbal, and just the overall lifestyle that these people lived were mind blowing. I dabbled with trumpet lessons in fifth grade and was asked to follow it through at least until sixth grade by the

gentleman at my elementary school who attempted to give me lessons. The horn didn't come as easily to me as I would have expected,
and I rapidly became bored with it. I was embarrassed to practice at
home as well, which made matters worse.

And then, to top it all off, a few weeks after school let out between
my last year of elementary school bliss and my first year of junior
high, my mother informed me that the marching band instruc-
tor called and wanted me to try it out for the summer. I remember
exactly what my stance was on this topic. "Listen, Mom, I love music,
but I suck at the trumpet! I can hardly play a basic scale on the
blasted thing!" I defended myself. "Well, then, what extracurricular
activities are you going to participate in once you get to junior high
school?" she questioned. I immediately spouted off, "What I'm good
at, which is tennis and skiing." "Listen, Jonathan, your dad and I both
know that you don't have any interest in a majority of the sports that
your friends excel at, and furthermore, skiing and tennis don't shift
into full throttle until winter and spring. Why don't you just go try it
out?" My mother usually has a good sense of intuition about decisions of this nature. She further coerced me by offering to purchase
a brand-new horn so that I didn't have to use one of the banged-up
band room loaners (which didn't help my playing technique a bit,
yet sure did make me look like I knew what I was doing in a Rodney
Dangerfield as Al Czervik, *Caddyshack* sort of way). After a couple
evenings of her pleading, I finally gave in and told her that I would
go check it out. "Jesus," I thought, "now half of my summer thrill is
going to be interrupted by fucking marching band practice!" It was
far from what I had in mind when it came to an activity of choice, but
a few nice benefits seemed to fall into place from being a second
chair trumpetist. When I arrived at D. S. Keith Junior High School,
I found myself in a melting pot of peers who had grandiose knowledge of bands and genres that I had no idea existed to that point.
Fellow musicians were into a slew of music in acts both random and
mainstream. From a fellow trumpeter I was able to get my hands on
a cassette that was entitled *Nevermind* from this Seattle-based trio

called Nirvana, which blew my mind from the first time I slipped the cassette into my Sony Walkman and hit Play on a bus trip to a state marching band competition traveling to Kings Dominion in Virginia. I found others who sank themselves into bands such as Nine Inch Nails, Jane's Addiction, Black Sabbath, Fugazi, The Dead Milkmen, the Violent Femmes, and Hole.

Another perk that took shape was finding other angles by which to plagiarize and cheat off of my peers on the academic front since packs of us sat in the same classes together. This strategy really paid dividends throughout those three years as I recall. But the most grandiose advantage of being surrounded by bandmates was that it presented an extensive opportunity to commingle with a great pool of adolescent girls who were becoming quite desirable to my explorative and vivid mind. As with the homework play that I would pull off regularly, I suppose that I had an adequate balance of awkward charm and humor back then. A handful of girls seemed interested in me on more of an experimentation level (as in, wanted to be a little more than casual friends). And I must say that it was an awesome rush of anxiety kissing and playfully exploring the opposite sex. Without a doubt, this sort of experimentation far exceeded any sort of knowledge that I would retain in a classroom setting. We would seek out desolate and darkened hallways in between practice and sometimes seek out slightly more intimate wooded areas between the school grounds and the practice fields where I was permitted to become acclimated with my newfound allure in exploration of the female anatomy. Looking back on it now, the band was a good experience and I'm glad that I stuck with it for those three years. I was a lousy horn player who faked more notes than I actually played. What I did realize was that I had a knack for tempo, beat, and harmony. The instrument never really bonded with me. However, a bunch of fond memories and great friends came out of the experience. Joining the band even gave me a sense of military structure as well, which was quite an eye-opener from my typical heedless demeanor.

As I transitioned to high school, I focused on extracurricular activities that better suited my interests such as skiing, snowboarding, tennis, golf, and girls. The trumpet was stashed away in a cedar closet in my bedroom for a couple years without ever being played. I enjoyed music immensely, but the brass family would not be my calling as far as musical expression was concerned. I had different plans for that. I attempted to explain to my mother that I still wanted to explore my musical interests but felt that I would be more suited for an instrument such as the guitar. My internal logic was pretty straightforward and simple in that I was interested in bands, not being in "the band." However, she wasn't having it. She had been encouraging me to learn the piano for years, but I knew that that, too, would not take and would become a disastrous waste of money due to lack of interest. I wanted an instrument that was cool to play and bold sounding. She didn't think that I would take guitar lessons seriously. Though my snide comeback of "Well, what do you think I would take more of a liking to?" carried modest weight, she refused to crack. So, in the meantime, I would have to settle in pretending to strum on tennis racquets as guitars, hockey sticks as bass, and an old remote control as an improvised microphone for singing along to MTV and cassette tapes blaring out of my Sony analogue player in the confines of my below-deck bedroom.

I quickly fused my favorite genres of modern bands from the late eighties and early nineties, then spliced them with those of the sixties and seventies. My brain morphed into an encyclopedia of great musical knowledge, which opened the magnificent exposed vault of bands such as The Jimi Hendrix Experience, Cream, The Doors, Led Zeppelin, The Who, the Grateful Dead, The Velvet Underground, Bob Dylan, Beck, Neil Young, and a slew of other greats. Yet still, purchasing latest issues of *Rolling Stone* magazine to learn about these icons didn't cut it for me. I wanted a shot to learn the machine that was rapidly shaping these adolescent years of mine.

Seeing as how my parents were not going to fund this little project, I needed to take matters into my own hands while being clever in my approach. I knew that I could hawk my trumpet to the right buyer for the right price and my parents would never know the difference. I had not a lick of negotiation skills or economic understanding back then, but if I did my instrument homework correctly, I'd have just enough bread to pick up a used Stratocaster of some sort and possibly a small amplifier if the stars lined up correctly. I began spreading the word in the halls and amongst friends that I had a "barely used" (at last I was telling the truth) trumpet for sale. Within a few weeks, I had a buyer, and together, the kid and I agreed on a solid price of four hundred dollars, which I figured was roughly half of the purchase value. The transaction went down smoothly, and with cash in hand, I began to set my eyes on the prize. The legit Fender and Washburn guitar/amp combos in the local music stores were vastly out of my price range so I needed to take a different approach. I only knew one person who owned an electric guitar at the time, and that was my good friend from physics class, Melanie. She and I were a dynamic duo in that class, taking two blue ribbons in both the egg drop and "weight-supported toothpick bridge" contests. We were good friends all through school, sharing mutual music interests. She introduced me to various bands such as Bad Religion, NOFX, and Porno for Pyros back in the day.

Melanie and I partnered up often in classes, but in physics class our senior year we were a force to be reckoned with! For whatever reason, we always studied at her house where we would sneak cigarettes, listen to music, and complete our given assignments. Her dad had bought her a Kay B1-K161 hollow body electric guitar accompanied with a small Fender practice amplifier a couple years earlier, which she on occasion would pull out of her closet and serenade me with her knowledge of a few choppy chords and scales. I sort of got the drift that she wasn't all that into it. She never took lessons, hardly played it, and kept the sunburst beauty behind a closed closet door in her bedroom. One day I asked her if she had any interest in selling me her guitar and further mentioned that I had budgeted four hundred cash for the purchase. At first, she declined the offer saying that the instrument was a Christmas or birthday or whatever gift given to her by her parents. A few days later, though, I think the internal reasoning of four hundred bucks to an eighteen-year-old had some practicality, and the ring of short-term cash in hand started to weigh on her. She finally agreed to the acquisition a day or so later and we would settle up in the school parking lot after classes let out. We each smoked a cigarette in her car to commemorate the occasion and she was excited for me, knowing that the guitar and amp would be taken care of and loved.

I could hardly wait to get it home to try it out after tennis practice that evening. Once home, I was so excited that I ended up telling my mother about how the deal went down. She was not disappointed in me but rather a bit impressed on how I had negotiated the bargain. She knew I was never going to play that horn again, and somehow I had the street smarts to acquire the goods that I fancied without the financial assistance or advice of adults with means. I went downstairs to my bedroom smiling ear to ear as I unloaded the tool from its dust-layered case, hit the power switch, threw the strap over my left shoulder, then pressed the reverb effect button while listening in uneducated delight as the machine screamed and bellowed out indecipherable notes and fingerings on the fretboard.

Later on that evening, the house phone rang. My mother summoned me from the top of the stairs and I briskly shot up the stairs to retrieve the phone call. "Hello"? I spoke into the receiver. "Jonathan, it's Melanie." She sounded distraught. "Hey, what's going on?" I asked, assuming that the matter was school related. "I need the guitar back," she said, almost weeping. "What?" I said, confused. "My parents grounded me and want to know if I can get the guitar back," she said softly. I could tell that she was in her room and not wanting her parents to overhear the conversation. "We had a deal," I said, both confused and slightly agitated. "I know. Listen, they made me call you to get it back. We'll talk about it in class tomorrow." "All right," I told her, now even more confused. I hung up and headed back downstairs to further experiment with my new musical project that now might be confiscated due to lack of judgment.

The next morning in Mr. Musselman's third period physics class, Melanie and I sat beside each other as always. She looked exceptionally drained. "What the hell happened last night?" I asked. "I already spent the money," she mumbled. "Already? We just settled up less than sixteen hours ago," I said, dumbfounded. Moments later, right before class was called to order, she told me in detail what she did with the funds. "I bought an ounce of pot right after you left my car"—I had no clue as to what the size or scale of the score even meant—"and I bought my prom dress last night." She sounded painfully resentful. "I'm grounded anyway so I really don't give a fuck," she added. And that was that! I thought surely that I would have to give the guitar back, especially if parents got involved. But when you buy a load of illegal contraband . . . I don't know much about drug transactions, but I don't think that dealer refunds at parents' demands are in the cards. Looking back, that is exactly how I would have wanted my first guitar transaction (out of several) to go down. Melanie confirmed that she did in fact get grounded for quite a spell and her parents didn't know the half of it! There were no hard feelings between us after the dust had settled. I still visited her house to work on school projects, and her folks approved of me. We set some extremely high bars in terms of physics projects, and our classroom marks reflected our efforts. We were both entrepreneurs in our own right as far as I saw it!

9

HARVARD

Listen, let's just call a spade a spade here. At some point, in my senior year of high school, I knew I had to start looking into what collegiate institution I would attempt to enroll in, thus extending my prodigious educational journey. My SAT scores were a slight train derailment of catawampus complexity in that the math section was borderline horrendous while my reading comprehension and writing were above average. After you'd tally up the points for simply signing your name to the top sheet on a two-try vault, my final score ended up somewhere around the one-thousand-point mark (which in all honesty impressed the shit out of me, knowing my academic track record).

Another key point before moving forward is that we all knew that there was no reason to waste the time or application fees on lavish schools that I didn't have a prayer of getting into. Point being that institutions such as Drexel, Franklin and Marshall, Duquesne, Villanova, Carnegie Mellon, and Bucknell were out of the question. So we needed to plan my odds-of-acceptance strategy accordingly. A realistic option (which I was not a huge fan of, by the way) was to apply to Penn State University, where I could attend two years at the nearby branch campus in Altoona completing my general education requirements. Then I could transition to the University Park campus in State College to finish out the major coursework to obtain my bachelor's degree. The positive was that there would be a handful of peers from high school as well as other local public schools who would be attending in the fall semester. The negative being, well, there was no downside after they accepted my application. It all made sense and that was that!

At the end of my senior year of high school, I realized that my initial thought to continue my education starting off at the Penn State Altoona campus was the correct play. It may not have been the perfect scenario at the time, but if nothing more, it would give me basic discipline and structure, as well as an automatic network of friends to pal around with.

As the beginning of my first semester approached, I naturally feared that the same academic struggles I'd battled for twelve years would resurface and crush my confidence. Even though I was living at home, I was still required to attend all freshmen introduction activities a week before classes began. I went through the motions and had a warm feeling that each and every one of us was now in the same camp. They did that drill (same as mentioned earlier with the sales training) where everyone stood in a straight line, looked to the right, then left, then the undergrad in charge would explain that it was likely the person beside you would not graduate due to a multitude of unforeseen reasons. It was a guilt tactic bestowed on the group that actually had some torque to it as I look back.

Those first two years, I truly hunkered down and applied myself the best that I could. I no longer could fault professors for not seeing eye to eye with my values. I realized that these people gave less than a shit about my academic fate unless I showed effort and spoke up about concerns. Somehow, I began to figure out the equation on how to get good grades and retain a majority of the material that was presented. This was mind blowing to me simply because, up to this point, I typically had the mindset that I was behind the eight ball and would have to kick desperately to keep my head above water to maintain average marks. The whole college environment had a vastly different feel, as I saw it. You could pick your own classes, find out from your peers and advisors which classes and professors you should choose, and if you were especially strategic in your approach, you'd line up classes with your friends so that you could study and commute to campus together.

Then at some point you start to understand that there is a massive financial element that comes into play (in my case, for my parents). All of this wasn't simply continuing education to pass time. Rather, you have to take a step back and find a general path and direction that you want to pursue. It became a great game of sorts. I started to understand how empowering it felt to set and hit goals. My attendance was near perfect and the subject matter was engaging, for the most part. Over my entire college career, I never once missed an eight o'clock class, I'm proud to say. And trust me, I skipped my share of classes throughout my tenure at Penn State University, but it was different than before. I didn't feel trapped, and figured out quickly that if I showed effort to my professors (in most any course and scenario) we could usually come up with some type of arrangement to benefit my case.

Wrapping up my first semester, I wound up with two As, two Bs, and a blasted C (due to a ridiculous anthropology class that I picked up as an elective, then realized that the material was way over my head. I never learned that you have the option to "late drop" a certain number of classes if you figure out within a couple weeks that the subject of choice turns out to be problematic for one reason or another). Yet that's water under the bridge at this point. Anyway, I was pretty impressed with what I pulled off. Between school, work, friends, guitar lessons, and snowboarding, it all felt as if I were gaining traction. Granted, it wasn't all perfect. I still struggled with certain areas of coursework, especially in my core courses. I enjoyed the business management, psychology, and marketing courses immensely while the struggle with algebra and economics persisted. I learned that the beautiful word "curve" was a fabulous perk and it saved me on many occasions.

* * *

A new advisor was assigned to me during my sophomore year and I set up an appointment to meet with him. I needed to declare a major as I was to transfer to Penn State University Park to start my junior year. This guy was great! He immediately sensed what I excelled at and where my weaknesses lay. He came up with a brilliant academic strategy, which, when I heard it, my gut reaction hollered, "Absolutely not!" Yet once he spelled out the path on paper, the logic behind it made perfect sense. "You want to get into a major focusing on business management, correct?" I did. "How does calculus sit with you, then?" he asked. "I'd rather have a broken back in hell," I immediately thought. "How about Applied Physics?" he inquired. "I'd rather be forced to see U2 (I despise U2) live before being dipped into a vat of boiling oil," bounced around in my head. "That's exactly what I figured," he confirmed. He told me that my best bet was to major in Hotel, Restaurant, and Recreational Management. At first, I about fell out of my chair. But then it was all made clear. "It's not so much about the major that you select, but rather getting the piece of paper at the finish line showing that you hit your goal," he explained. In other words, "Just get a degree and the rest will figure itself out!" It was a freaking brilliant angle to see my future! "You don't have to know what you want to be when you grow up," he said. "Discipline and the ability to set goals are the key to finding what one is passionate about." It wasn't that I was preparing myself to become a housekeeping manager at the Hyatt Regency or the next food and beverage director at the Wynn in Las Vegas. Then again, having options is always a good thing!

The guy even gave me a stock tip on an algebra professor for the following semester to fulfill the dreaded math requirements needed. The only drawback was that the class was held once a week on Saturdays at a three-hour clip. Though the thought of this was flat-out atrocious, he assured me that the guy was extremely fair so long as effort and attendance were applied. Naturally, I took his advice and bit the bullet that semester. When the dust settled, I received a B minus, which was nothing short of a spectacular grade-curving miracle.

As my two-year tenure was winding down in Altoona, I was excited to attend the University Park campus of Penn State. After two years of patiently waiting while still having the perks of cooked dinners and laundry detail at my beck and call, it was time to officially be on my own. A whole host of my friends, both old and new, were going up together, and I can't recall a one of us who wasn't chomping at the bit for the second chapter of our college experience to begin.

A couple of guys from the Bellmeade crew were leasing a townhouse with three other Altoona natives from the year before. One tenant was transferring to another school in the fall, so they asked me months before if I would like to fill the spot. It took little coaxing and thought to sway me into filling the vacancy. The apartment was located two miles from campus and fairly far out from the pandemonium and chaos of the downtown and campus area. It was quiet on that side of town. You didn't have to worry about paying for parking or dealing with the traffic congestion of the downtown area. These guys as a whole kept to themselves. They were studious, laid back, and mainly cared about hunting, fishing, smoking piles of cigarettes, drinking beer, and betting on sports through an anonymous Altoona bookie. For the most part, the group was not into socializing outside of our small clique, partying, or attending any sort of on-campus extracurricular functions. Hell, the entire complex was docile and a bit dismal for my liking. Neither here nor there. You went to class, got your schoolwork done. That's about all the frills that place had going for it. On weekends, those guys would get a bit rowdy watching sports, drinking beer, and smoking cigarettes until the packs and lungs were exhausted. I was neither a sports watcher nor a gambler nor a beer drinker back then, so I got busy finding alternate activities to waste my time when not studying.

The semester fell into swing, and even though a couple of my classes were going to be insanely difficult and require an enormous amount of time and effort, the academic balance began to take shape and I fell back into the groove just as I did in Altoona. However, a couple weekends after the semester set in, I found myself bored and pretty much discontented with my social environment. Sitting around playing guitar hours on end by myself in our bedroom and watching baseball with my roommates all afternoon wasn't exactly living up to the epic college experience that I'd dreamt up over the past two years.

* * *

In my next attempt to enhance my social network, I joined the club snowboard team and began to rush fraternities in the same week. I had little knowledge as to what this whole Greek system deal was all about, yet I had a few buddies from back home who'd had some great experiences pursuing these organizations. My issue was not the socializing aspect but rather the drinking component that everyone talked about. Alcohol simply wasn't my thing back then. I just didn't get it. Beer tasted like shit and I had just enough experience on the subject that my insides churned just thinking about a couple of pounding hangovers while trying to figure out what all of the hype was about. I came up with a script of sorts as I pursued different houses attempting to find the correct fit during a courting process more or less. These "ballers" would roll out the red carpet with all sorts of pathetic gimmicks to entice flocks of naive rushes by means of hosting "ornate" brotherhood events such as dinners and parties, or dinner parties or "happy hours," which always tended to end up with beer pong, thumping hip hop sounds, and a couple handfuls of random girls to enhance the overall effect of the atmosphere.

In conversations with these guys, I would be sure to explain my stance on alcohol and drugs with a clear message of intent as I winnowed my decision down to a couple of houses where I might consider pledging. "If I join and you guys force me to drink, I'm out!" That was my motto. And, for the most part, they all said that they respected my values on the subject. I truly was impressed by how many of these houses operated as recognized university entities. They were all involved in a plethora of activities both on campus and off, which was exactly what I was looking for. They hosted social gatherings and parties with neighboring fraternities while structuring events with sororities, which was right up my alley. All the while, the repeated theme was that, yes, there was a pledging process, but academic integrity remained the top priority with mandatory study hours and class attendance monitored closely by your pledge educator (an appointed position to a brother who was responsible for the pledge class). If this all held true, this was my ticket to the complete social experience, I thought. On the final weekend of rush, as a few bids were offered to me, I made my decision to pledge Alpha Kappa Lambda that fall semester.

Now it felt as if everything was in place. My days became overwhelmingly busy with classes, schoolwork, fraternity obligations, and getting involved in just about every event and activity that I could get into. I resumed my guitar lessons with a well-known and accomplished musician who lived close to the apartment. Once he felt I was comfortable with time, he even got me plugged in with a few jamming locals who periodically invited me to play rhythm guitar and sing backup vocals on a few songs while playing a happy hour at a local drinking establishment or a late-night open mic session. Getting involved was amazing! The guys back at the apartment thought that I was insane for taking all this on so quickly. With long days and most of my time now spent on campus and at the fraternity house, which was most conveniently located close to downtown, I began to grow distant from them. I formed a new core group of friends. My apartment mates weren't very impressed with either my lifestyle or the three-o'clock-in-the-morning phone calls that woke up the entire compound (cell phones were just becoming a "thing" at that point) with any random brother calling me with instructions to report to the house at once for random detail. I got the message.

Time passed with a sense of structure that I was comfortable with. My classes were becoming much more demanding as I got into my core 300- and 400-level classes. As before, I struggled with certain classes such as Advanced Accounting and Statistics but was very engaged in most others. It was a juggling act of sorts trying to balance my academic obligations and extracurricular activities. I took on an internship the following summer with the Altoona Curve minor league baseball team working as an assistant to the food and beverage manager. The experience was great, but the commute back and forth was anything but ideal.

Going into my senior year, I was spread extremely thin with my course load, but I needed a certain amount of "industry hours," which were required upon graduation. Once my internship requirements were completed at the ballpark, I took on another part-time job at the on-campus hotel called The Nittany Lion Inn. I'm not sure to this day how I landed the gig, but they made me a server in the lounge and bar operation. The hotel was one of the fancier establishments in the area, and the lounge—properly called "Whiskers" after the school mascot Nittany Lion—was known as a hobnobbing drinking establishment for middle- and upper-class patrons. My dad was especially proud that I'd landed the position. This was one of his favorite joints in the area to pony up to the elaborate oak bar, grab a few brews of his liking, and engage in conversation with whomever walked through the door and posted up beside him.

I figured out the trade pretty quickly via a few veteran staff members, and in no time, the hustle was on! Shortly thereafter, my manager asked if I was interested in learning the bartending trade. Of course I was! I learned to mix up highbrow cocktails such as choice bourbon old-fashioned, martinis, manhattans, and sidecars along with knowledge of an extensive wine list that made the pickings ripe for high-dollar ticket amounts. The result was aligning gratuities. When you combine a great cast of fellow coworkers with some nice loot in your pocket at the end of a shift, the experience was awesome. The only part that I would have changed looking back was my financial awareness at that time. Purchasing guitars, amplifiers, four-track recorders, synthesizers, microphones, and piles of compact discs was all that was on my mind back then. In hindsight, I would have fared far better if I had saved rather than spend in semi-erratic behavior. I suppose that I was young and didn't understand the value of a dollar as I do today. Regardless, this was such a simple and yet amazing time when I look back on it.

The following semester, I decided to move out of the apartment and take up residency in the fraternity house. It simply made sense. I sensed that those guys were tired of my shit. I was there only to sleep by that point. Time had run its course there and it was best for me to find a dwelling that better suited my lifestyle.

I also started dating a girl from California, whom I had met randomly during an internship that I had acquired at the Altoona minor league baseball stadium. This girl was eighteen going on thirty-seven from a maturity standpoint. She carried herself with an exact sway straight out of Santa Monica with the body and brashness to go with it. To set the record straight, she was completely out of my league and barely out of high school. The positive was that she attended an all-girls private school in the area, so fortunately there was really no bar set for her at that point. This girl gave me an education and outlook on life that was in and of itself worthy of a graduate degree— from sex and drug experimentation to being world traveled thanks to a posh and entitled upbringing. She also had no hesitation in contesting authority. She was like no personality that I had ever met to that point. Sure, I had been in a handful of semi-serious relationships, but this girl obliterated any trace of purity that was left in my ever-inquisitive body. And yet she was somehow intrigued by my charm and preposterous sense of humor.

She would be attending college in Baltimore in the fall, so of course we tried our hand at the long-distance relationship angle, which, considering our ages, was destined to fail. But while they lasted, our adventures were always epic in terms of unsupervised worldliness to the ninth degree in unchartered waters. We then decided to sublet an apartment for the summer in State College until classes resumed for the fall semester. This seemed like a brilliant idea, as we had planned it all out. Then, about halfway through the summer, well, let's just say that the honeymoon period of ten months had run its course and slammed straight into a brick wall (quite literally as you'll see in just a moment). Fighting, fucking, yelling, breaking up, making up, and getting back together were all part of the equation in those few blissful months. I once recall her pulling a random bottle of beer out of the refrigerator one night and firing it off the brick wall in our bedroom after accusing me of taking notice of an attractive co-ed earlier that day. The bottle naturally exploded upon impact sending shards of glass and ale everywhere at three o'clock in the morning in a fit of rage. In turn, I waited until she left for work the next morning, cleaned up the remainder of the glass from the prior evening's tantrum, and shoved a bag full of clothes, guitars, and microphones into the trunk of my Subaru. I stopped at the local convenience store to grab two packs of cigarettes and four Mountain Dews, and then bolted for the beach to join my family on vacation at the Delaware shore for the week.

One thing that I realized rather quickly is that I didn't need to take shit like this from anybody. Did I feel bad about any of it, you may ask? Not in the least! I'd learned through years of being hollered at by my father that the best tactic in a one-sided argument is, as the receiver, to put your head down and take the verbal assault while allowing the perpetrator's words to slide in one ear and out through the other, paying no mind to the subject matter at hand. You should not speak unless told to do so. Let the person vent. I was becoming pretty darn accomplished in simmering down altercations, and in this specific case, my actions struck a far deeper nerve than any choice words in a heated moment. Needless to say, after a year or so, the relationship was falling apart. I did my part in driving her back to school once her classes were to start again. She was dropped off at a friend's house in a suburb of Baltimore where we exchanged a final embrace and I sped off back to State College. A few weeks went by before we finally spoke again. A small but weak case was made to rekindle the relationship that evening. A few of my close buddies from the house swayed me into breaking the relationship off for good. So, that's what I did with a good, old-fashioned broken-voiced phone call. Yes, of course, the act hurt quite a bit, and then the heartbroken absence set in hard in the aftermath of it all. But it was a necessary move at the time.

10

TEN-SECOND NEWS

A few weeks prior to the "Little Miss Cali hurls bottle off the wall" incident, my mother called to inform me that they were taking our annual family summer trip to the Delaware shore. She wanted to know of my plans and if I intended to drive down for any or all of the week's festivities. I told her that with our work schedules in the service industry and all that it was going to be tough to swing a jaunt to the beach that year. She understood my logic in the matter, and we caught up with other goings-on. Now, granted, I talk to my mom pretty much every few days, so it's never as if there are weeks of news to catch up on. That particular afternoon, I was at the apartment by myself and I could tell that something was off in our conversation. She made a one-off statement that went something to the effect of, "That's perfectly fine that you can't come to the shore; it's just that we could really use your help this year." A passive/

aggressive tone began to develop that was extremely out of character for her. A couple more off-kilter comments were made. Finally, I stopped the dialogue and simply asked, "Mom, what's going on with you today?"

She paused for roughly three seconds to catch her breath and construct her thoughts. Then she began, her tone collapsing, "It's your dad. He's sick, Jonathan. I mean really, really sick." I was both inquisitive as well as perplexed. "With what?" I asked. "He has had a few episodes over the past months and we got him to a doctor last week. I didn't want you three to know just in case everything checked out for the good. Well, It didn't. They found a large mass on the right front temporal lobe of his brain. We found out yesterday that it is malignant."

I was trying my best to absorb each word. "So what does that mean?" I tried to remain positive. "Jonathan, your father has brain cancer." At this point, she broke down. "Well, what can they do to treat it?" I asked. "They are going to begin radiation next week in an attempt to shrink the tumor. Once the first round of treatments is over, they will reevaluate and tell us what our options are," my mother told me. "How is he feeling?" I asked. "He has good days and bad days. He has no headaches and feels no pain. He does have periodic episodes where he can't process motor skills. One morning last week, he spent almost an hour trying to put his socks and shoes on." "How long have you noticed these spells going on?" I asked. "They've become more frequent over the past six weeks. I knew something was seriously wrong."

While she began giving me details of my father's strange behavior over the past several weeks, an incident crossed my mind from two months ago. Katie and I were home from school for Easter where we did the typical go-to-church-in-the-morning followed by family-coming-over-for-a-big-lunch spread in the afternoon. It was a typical after-church Sunday for us. I was casually getting my belongings together to head back to school before it became too late. Typically, my dad would be involved in ten tasks at a time barking orders while cooking, cleaning, all while simultaneously tending to a house project or washing a vehicle. After the company had left, I noticed him sitting on an old wooden rocking chair in the living room. I had never seen anyone, let alone him, sit on that piece of furniture—it was a decorative piece of my mom's and certainly not a La-Z-Boy intended for comfort. He sat there for an absurdly long amount of time, not rocking in relaxation but simply sitting there motionless with a blank stare on his face as the typical family chaos ensued around him. I did not hear him speak, and his face was completely expressionless as if he were staring off into space, remaining deep in thought. It was just uncharacteristic of him. Perhaps he was simply exhausted, or had a lot on his mind at work and he was basking in his family all being home for the Easter holiday. In the days that followed, I told my mother of this observation. And as we started to put the pieces together, she agreed immediately that this was certainly in line with what she had witnessed firsthand over the past couple of months.

"Well, why would you go on vacation if he's not well?" I questioned, over the phone. "We think it would be best to get him away for a few days," she replied. "Besides, your aunt and uncle will be down there to help out if we run into any problems. He has more good days than bad right now, but that may change once he begins his radiation treatments." The logic made sense to me. I assured her that I would come home in the next few days so she could further debrief me and we could generate some sort of game plan to prepare for the next few months.

* * *

When I got home a few days later, I was relieved to see my father energetic and in good spirits. He was only permitted to go into work a couple of days per week for just a few hours a day. He was aware that he was sick, yet to what degree I hadn't a clue. He was given stern instruction from his doctors not to drive unless necessary. My mom was in the final year of gaining her doctorate degree from Penn State as well so I knew that her juggling act between my dad, her day job, her studies, and other household goings-on would become a noticeable setback through this whole ordeal. Katie was to spend the summer at the beach with her friends. When news hit that Dad was diagnosed, she was forced to change her plans and stay home for the summer. We tried to be selective as to what we shared with Makenzie for the time being, fearing that it was a bit much for her to understand at the age of thirteen. My grandparents returned home from Florida so that my grandfather could assist my uncle in running the daily operation of the business while my dad was not present. Our entire family dynamic was starting to shift as the weeks passed, and Dad started his first round of radiation treatments shortly after Memorial Day. He lost his hair and grew weak as a result of the radiation. I would joke with him that he looked like Mr. Clean the first time that I walked into the house and saw him with no hair. I always tried to keep the mood light when I would come home. A few times, I would occasionally take him to the local hospital in Altoona for his treatments, which lasted forty-five minutes to an hour. In his typical fashion, he knew the entire staff at the treatment clinic within a week. On visits to and from, I don't recall us ever talking about him being sick. He fell into a routine of hospitals and doctors and other medical appointments while remaining positive through the entire process. My mom and friends in the medical industry arranged for second opinions through larger networks such as Johns Hopkins in Baltimore in an effort to understand all the options available when dealing with an inoperable tumor. She sought out nutritionists who would focus on balancing his diet to fight the cancer from the inside out. All tactics and means to cancer treatment were taken into consideration.

In May, my mom received her doctorate from Penn State. We celebrated at Whiskers (naturally) after the commencement was over. Dad was super proud that day and in great spirits. I'll never forget that. But as the summer months eventually melted into fall, you could see the sick in his eyes. Always an avid runner, his balance and muscle control deteriorated rapidly—that was hard for me to witness.

We did our best to keep him comfortable and upbeat. My family agreed that it was for the best that no plans be altered for the family vacation that summer in Delaware (the vacation that I was not planning on attending because of my work schedule). Everyone needed a break and my dad loved it down there.

So, on that bat-shit crazy evening in the apartment, which I mentioned a few moments ago, as bottles of ale were whizzing past my head, it may have been a sign from God that my family needed me there to help out with Dad rather than dealing with this sort of domestic lunacy. And that was the moment that I devised the plan to bolt as soon as she left for work the next morning. When I reached the Delaware shore hours later, I saw that my mother's intuition had been accurate three months prior when she'd told me about Dad's cancer and that they could use my help down there this year. My uncle Frank had driven them all down a few days before I'd arrived. I hadn't seen Dad for around a week at that point. My dad was in rough shape when I got there. He was extremely confused by his surroundings. His fine motor skills were affected. We had to help him put his clothes on and assist him with using utensils while he ate. During the evenings, Uncle Frank and I would sit with him around the fire laughing and carrying on as if nothing had changed. Then the two of us would help him into the camper where my mother, Aunt Judy, my uncle, and I would get him ready for bed and make him feel comfortable for sleep. Then Uncle Frank and I would go back out and resume our talks and catch up as the evening set in. These were extremely emotional conversations as I look back on those fireside chats. I have always looked up to my Uncle Frank like no other. But this time he was unable to give me the practical advice like he always did in the past. His voice cracked several times as he fought back tears. He was rapidly losing his brother-in-law as well as best friend.

* * *

You could feel the toll that cancer was taking on my family. In the ensuing months, an outpouring of prayers, cards, and love from friends, associates, and loved ones began to cascade around us. The following month, Dad's equilibrium and basic motor skills became impacted. He went from the use of a cane to a walker to a wheelchair. Doctors were still administering radiation treatments, but all of us around him saw that the poison was making him weak. Family, friends, and neighbors would stop by throughout the day to visit and drop off meals and offer assistance to my mother when they could.

I began staying at home a couple nights a week at this point to help my mom out. Luckily, my employers were extremely understanding of my situation and cut my hours. It was around this time that we were informed Dad's radiation treatments were to be suspended until further notice. He spent most days in bed and we would transition him to his wheelchair so that he wouldn't have to spend the entire day there. His voice and speech started to become weak and scrambled. He would become confused mid-sentence, not being able to finish his thoughts. He would compensate by using two- or three-word statements in a whisper. We'd get him showered and freshened up as best we could. His limbs risked atrophy as he spent more and more time resting in bed. He was barely able to stand on trips to the bathroom, his legs shaking with intense spasticity. We would all take turns at his bedside talking to him. He was usually conscious, but his sense of being alert to his surroundings was dwindling.

School for all three of us kids began in late August. I was in my senior year, Katie was a sophomore at Slippery Rock University north of Pittsburgh, and Makenzie was going into eighth grade in junior high. I was going to be diving into fifteen credits consisting mainly of 400-level core courses. Upon the start of the fall semester, I was tactical, very quickly making all of my professors aware of my situation. No doctor's note or proof of reason was needed upon explanation! The professors all knew my family had a dire set of circumstances on our hands. I was able to balance out the beginning of the year to the best of my ability. Getting home at beck and call was rather simple. Katie, on the other hand, was three hours away. As she heard of Dad's rapidly declining condition, she withdrew from the fall semester of her sophomore year and headed home.

At a certain point in the days to come, my mother lined up a social worker to come by the house and give recommendations as to what our options were. She then sat me down to discuss the situation at length. Between eating, transferring from bed to chair, changing diapers, bathing, and so many other daily tasks, we wanted Dad to be comfortable when the time came. Especially for my youngest sister's sake, I was not on board with a hospice service coming in to the house to care for him in his final days. We both agreed that he should not pass in his home. So, we made the decision to admit him into the palliative care unit at the Altoona hospital. This decision was for the best and we both knew it. My father's fate was out of our control now.

The social worker returned the following day and the arrangements were made. I took Makenzie down to my bedroom and explained to her as best I could what was going to happen later that afternoon. "The ambulance workers are going to come get Dad and take him to the hospital today. They will take really good care of him there. Much better than we can do here until he gets better. OK?" This was the gist of explaining the situation to my thirteen year old kid sister. I gave her a hug and she was tough as nails when the ambulance pulled down our driveway that afternoon.

The mood was certainly heavy that day as the team transferred Dad from his bed to the stretcher. I distinctly told Makenzie to just stay down in my room until they all left, but I think her curiosity got the best of her as she saw her father being taken away from the home in which he'd spent countless days bricklaying, restoring, and remodeling. She started to cry when she saw them wheeling him through the house and into the ambulance. There were no sirens or lights, no rushing to the destination at hand for emergency medical treatment. The EMS team was very professional and courteous. There was no fanfare in the transport. They did their job and were soon on their way.

I had to go back to school the night that he was admitted but would return the next evening to visit him in the hospital. And this is how it went in the days thereafter. I would wake up, go to class, head for the hospital, spend time with my dad, study, and either return to the fraternity house or go home to sleep. With Dad out of the house, the pressure of twenty-four-hour care was now lifted off of my mother, and I felt good about that. Having a household transform into a one-person hospital over the past couple of months had left its scar as I would pace through our home in disbelief, typically when everyone else was at the hospital. The now useless medical devices, wheelchair, wellness books, stacks of unopened bills and cards, and that overbearing smell of hospital latex and medicine still lingered.

Sitting through class was challenging. I realized immediately that it was best that Katie had come home when she did. It was extremely difficult to focus. I did my best not to take advantage of the flexibility that my professors offered with my attendance and coursework. I cried often while walking on campus, wearing sunglasses to hide my tears. Text messaging was in its infancy at that point, so acquiring on-demand updates from my family was nearly impossible. I would ponder all day how I would feel if I wasn't present when the time came to say goodbye. I'd race along back roads to get to the hospital, then brace myself in the elevator on the way up to the fourteenth floor as to what news I would receive upon entering the palliative care unit. As somber of a wing that it was, all the nurses were great. "No change," or "He's still hanging in there" would be mentioned by staff before I would enter his room, and a sense of relief would suffuse through me.

The sights and sounds that one would hear on a typical hospital floor were nonexistent on this level. No machines to monitor heart rate, no IV stands or defibrillators around. The whole unit was made up of a central common space that looked like a lounge area of a priority pass executive club in an airport, yet with a somber, quiet library feel. Several couches, tables, and desks with telephones were arranged properly with six or so rooms that lined the perimeter on either end. Professionals would flow in and out in a soft manner from time to time to check on patients and report updates to family members and loved ones.

I would immediately bounce into his room and give him a huge hug and a kiss on the top of his head. I would thank him for holding the fort down while I was gone. At times, he was awake and alert. There were no feeding tubes or wires or medical machinery of any sort. I would prop myself up on the edge of his bed. There, I'd hold his hand and talk to him for as long as I could. "It's Ok to let go. You don't have to be afraid to leave us. I'll take care of everything. We all love you so much," was repeated over and over and over again each day.

One of those days, I arrived at the hospital early. He seemed to be more alert than in days prior. I took his hand and started talking to him. He slowly positioned his head to look out the window, then back at me. He did this several times as we caught up on whatever was on my mind. I told him that I loved him so much. And, a moment later, he readjusted his hand as if to apply a stronger pressure to his grip. He looked at me directly with those painfully sick, bloodshot eyes, and in a whisper of all the strength he could gather, he said, "I love you, pal." I blasted into tears, yet they were good tears. He hadn't spoken a coherent sentence in days from what I was told. My mom was not going to believe this!

As the weekend approached, we were simply in a holding pattern. Friends and acquaintances from all over came to visit with him. I remember it was a bit chaotic for staff at times because guests lined up in the corridors outside, but we let most everyone who wanted to spend a few moments with him do so. Gifts and flower arrangements and catered dinners poured in to that unit at all hours of the day.

As that weekend set in, I brought enough essentials down with me to camp out on the fourteenth floor until I had to return to class the following Monday. By this point, we had each shed our tears and said our goodbyes. We all figured that the end of this odyssey was almost upon us. The couches were plush enough to sleep on so

I brought a pillow. I could study and catch up on my coursework; the staff even permitted me to bring up one of my acoustic guitars so long as I played softly in the evening when no one was around. (For whatever reason, I remember learning the song "Satellite" by the Dave Matthews band up there because I could finger-pick the notes at a piano volume softness without disturbing the couple of occupied rooms around me.)

Saturday passed without incident. Katie and I got into the routine of "sneaking" out a rear entrance of the building exit to suck down packs of cigarettes. The term "visiting hours" did not apply to us by this point. We simply killed time as best we could. On Sunday morning, a heightened activity level on the unit stirred me at some point in the morning. Moments later, someone (I cannot remember who in my groggy state of mind) exclaimed, "Jonathan, let's go— its time!" I rocketed up off the couch and headed for the room. I specifically remember that one of my dad's great friends, Rodney (Bummy) Baumgartner, had dropped by to visit that morning. With all the commotion going on, he realized that his timing was off. In the room, my entire family had gathered around Dad's bed. I positioned myself on the far side where I could squeeze in to be near him up toward the top of the bed. A nurse entered the room and gave a brief explanation as to what to expect. She explained very calmly that he would begin to convulse, his body taking multiple seizures until it was over. His breathing became sporadic, weak, and extremely irregular. Within moments, a paralyzing seizure took hold of him. His red eyes rolled to the back of his head as the spasticity again shook his entire body, lasting approximately a minute. Finally, as a smaller shock wave set in, he seemed to be choking on his own breath. His entire body began to collapse inwards. And with one small remaining choking breath, it was over. His life had ended.

The room collapsed in an overwhelming state of sorrow. Everyone took their turn to express remorse and say their farewells. Several minutes after, the room thinned out until only my mother and I remained hovering over my father's lifeless body. Very little was said between us as I went to her. I held her as she sobbed in disbelief. Shortly after, I left the room to give her the time she needed. Back in the lounge area, several people were crying and hugging. I passed through the crowd and made my way to a window in the corner of the room to gather my thoughts. On a spectacularly sunny day, I looked out over my hometown. I was not crying. I was simply numb.

Funeral arrangements were made, and the outpouring of sympathy and love for my father and our family were of staggering proportion. After all affairs were back to some sort of basic order at home, I needed to shift gears immediately back to academics. I was a little behind, but the deficit was manageable. I got back on track and even began to pick up shifts again at Whiskers. It was a nice feeling to simply be a student again, which reminds me: The guys at the fraternity were extremely supportive of my situation as well. My dad got to know a handful of these collegiate clowns from football tailgates as well as other organized events over the years. A whole slew of these friends made the drive and were in attendance for all of my dad's services. It truly meant so much to me at the time. That entire semester was a complete whirlwind on so many different levels. Even though it felt great to be back amongst my peers, there was still a void. I worried about my mom and Makenzie a lot. I didn't attend a single football game, which in our realm was considered an act of blasphemy. Working and playing guitar were two relaxing outlets for me during that period of time. Keeping to myself was another by-product of my grieving, and those who know me know that this was extremely atypical behavior on my part. I blamed no one for the events that happened over the previous months. God needs my father in heaven more than I need him here was a constant thought that I pondered as the wounds began to heal. I learned to accept that.

That semester, I received a 3.5 GPA, which blew my fucking mind! Yeah, I believe that there may have been a few sympathy tweaks in my grading calculation from a few understanding professors, but my dad would have been so proud of me when I got my grades at the end of that semester. I gave God the angel that he asked for. In turn, he did me one solid on the grading curve. You made out pretty well on that return, Big Guy!

For whatever reason, the manner by which my courses played out put me a semester behind, which I learned is a quite common revenue generation tactic for universities and colleges. It becomes nearly impossible to graduate in a given four years unless substantial coursework loads and summer school balance out the equation at the end of the game. That formula wasn't going to work in my graduation strategy, as I was taking classes over the summer to get professors who tended to be more lax in their syllabus structure. Courses such as Accounting 420, Statistics 202, Economics 320, and Labor and Industrial Relations 350 were all roadblocks that needed to be detoured through summer sessions to ensure an adequate average. And this was fine by me because, in all honesty, here was my situation: I enjoyed my current quality of life as a student, I had no clue as to what I wanted to be when I grew up, my tuition and boarding was on my mother's dime, and I knew that I could play the "dead dad" card for a while to pass time until graduation. So, I made the absolute most out of the given situation.

Somewhere through this all, I realized that the complete college experience consisted roughly of 50 percent academic knowledge and 50 percent of the social surroundings that make up your experience. My academic finish line was in the foreseeable future and well within reach at this point. Deceleration was not an option on the academic front; however, self-experimentation in my surroundings was an opportunity that I was going to indulge myself in. So much time was spent fretting about making grades and dropping out and failing that I really didn't embrace the whole vision back then. Failure would have likely been unavoidable if I would have thrown myself into the bucket headfirst as some of my peers did. But I elected to take the road of slow, steady, and cautious. So that's how I played the hand (with one exception).

My final semester at Penn State University was a peaceful protest of anarchism none to what I was used to. The way that the year

played out, I had four credits remaining plus finishing out my industry hour requirements, which would be a breeze. A far more reserved
and withheld personality of a few years prior shed a layer of skin
that was a pertinent final step before the chapter of professionalism
to come. Let's just say that I lived a lifestyle akin to that of Jim Mor-
rison. Partying, girls, dabbling in drugs and hard alcohol, music, and
petty larceny were all in the cornucopia of young adult freedom and
expression. The behavior that I should have been expressing as a
freshman or back in high school, for that matter, was now surfacing.
Through friends in the local music scene, I started sharing ideas with
fellow musicians. Impromptu jams in apartments became legit practices became trial happy hours became full-blown shows at local
watering holes throughout State College and surrounding areas. Performing solo and in duo acoustic acts for the most part was a great
stepping-stone as I managed to find my sea legs playing your typical
cover numbers in front of locals, hoped-up students, and friends, but
having the opportunity to collaborate with various talents on the
local scene was a real eye-opener.

On guitar, my skill level was far off from having any type of particular style, but performing with others who had the experience of
playing with full four- to five-piece acts was an absolute blast. I had
absolutely no sort of stage presence to speak of, nor did any of us
dubs need one for all intents and purposes. What they did appreciate was my octave range, steady rhythm playing, working through
complex harmony parts, and the completely obscure catalog of
songs that I brought to the table when working out new arrangements. I was open to it all—punk, blues, hip-hop, and anything trend-
ing that sounded worthwhile at the time. The creative freedom of
merging, let's say, a typical David Bowie number with a set of Snoop
Dogg lyric plugs in the bridge, then some sort of jam outro, would
have been a completely acceptable number when the parts lined up
correctly. I learned all sorts of lead guitar hooks and tricks as well
as improved my skill set. This group of comrades would play typically Thursday through Saturday at just about any spot that would

shovel out a hundred bucks plus the door for driving in patrons. No one really cared about making any serious bread off of these shows. More times than not, the earnings were given back to the house at the end of the night to pay soundboard staff and late-night bar tabs far after our free drink period was expunged. It was an incredible period of time! We would stay up all hours of the night raising holy hell and jamming and sleeping in until noon to do it all again the next day. We would crash at each other's houses and apartments to keep a late-night shindig going even though we lived mere minutes away from each other, and we'd wake up with guitars and amplifiers and girls and gear spread out all over the couches and floors.

As this rambunctious lunacy continued weekend after weekend, the semester as well as my college experience was finally drawing to a close. As previously stated, my final semester was a breeze. I scheduled my final meetings with my academic advisor to be sure that my affairs were in order. Everything checked out. Jonathan Miller was going to graduate! Now, granted, I hadn't the faintest clue as to what I was going to embark on professionally in the next chapter of my life, but I had faith that I would figure it out in due time. And an important mindset started to fall into place. The golden and yet frightening question of "Where do you truly see yourself in five years?" began to set in. All around me, my friends were graduating and going off to new careers and adventures. My reality was completely up in the air. I needed to get out of this area to find my path and myself. My life seemed very coddled with somewhat of a spoiled upbringing to this point. And yet, what was to be expected, honestly? My father was handed a business with a bank roll from my grandfather's entrepreneurial intuition, my mother hadn't paid for a vehicle or a tank of gasoline since she was wed, we three children were gifted with vehicles and exquisite vacations, and none of us owed a dime of student debt upon graduation from our respective universities (thanks to our mother's firm belief in a strong education for all of her children).

The year before Dad got sick, my grandfather approached me and asked if I had any desire in joining the family business. I respectfully declined, knowing in my gut that the current wholesale florist business model would not be sustainable long term, as technology and larger competition would eventually undercut and absorb the smaller operations such as ours. I watched how hard my father had to work in an environment that he was never passionate about but that had made sense when he was young. I had an entrepreneurial spark in me, and the family operation didn't feel like my calling. My outgoing personality and forward-thinking vision told me that I would make a good manager in the correct environment if I were passionate about the cause. I enjoyed devising business plans and operational strategies. A pact of sorts started to devise in my head. The goal was to start my own venture before the age of thirty. This gave me a cushion of eight years to figure out the particulars. Again, the details of all this were simply assumed. The location and financial structure were to figure themselves out. That was my plan of action.

As for those final moments as an undergrad, I was planning to do it up in spectacular fashion. So, that's just what I did. Commencement would be held the next week. The mood was a little bittersweet as I stepped up on that stage amongst those typical university types, keynote speakers, and my peers to receive my diploma. Though several of my family members were in attendance, my dad was not. My mom suggested that I carry his wedding band in my pocket to ensure that he was with me that day in spirit as I finally crossed the finish line.

11

LEAVING HOPE

Everything was hazy. Discomforting room sounds of beeping and buzzing were pounding through my head. People were talking above me and all around, but whether they were talking to me or about me or nothing to do with me was unclear. The multiple IV bags and tubes were barely visible from my vantage point, yet tubes ran in all directions to me or the table or bed, or whatever the hell I was lying on top of. Every few moments, the sound of a different machine triggered and rang out accordingly. A female nurse or doctor came over and put the back of her hand on my cheek cautiously as her face dissolved to a blurred silhouette. She spoke words, but I had no clue if they were directed at me or someone else. Whether I said or moaned or grunted anything in response, I hadn't a clue. There was so much to process in all the hustle of that environment.

The recollection of the anesthetist fixing me moments before was clear evidence that my memory was indeed in check. The surgery had happened! The number of times that my blurred vision faded in and out of consciousness is unknown, but it seemed very frequent. There was a pumping sort of sound generating from the bottom of the bed. Something attached to my legs would tighten excessively as the machine cranked on, and then the pressure would release moments later just to fill up again. People were attending to me in all directions. An automatic blood pressure machine on my right side turned on and spat out a reading. The entire environment felt slow with a non-stopping humming sound. Vision would set to focus temporarily, and then heavy lids followed by sudden exhaustion would push me down into darkness again.

Each time awaking, there were different sounds and a new cast of professionals tending to me. One person shined an insanely bright flashlight into my eyes back and forth repeatedly while another was applying some sort of ointment above my right eye. My body didn't move. It felt mummified while the machines around me carried out their specific functions. My neck could adjust only a couple inches from side to side as the urge to process my surroundings took priority between blackouts. The feeling was extremely agitating and beyond uncomfortable. More refined grunts and groans started to develop as my preferred means of communication during what could have been minutes or possibly days. That professional woman kept appearing, trying to communicate something, but the intense buzzing sound in my ears prevented me from interpreting any of her mouth movements precisely. A tingling in my nose developed. An attempt was made to carefully lift one of my arms to my face to relieve the annoyance. However, both arms remained fixed to the bed upon my attempt to raise them. "These bastards have me restrained!" I thought in disbelief. Yet perhaps this was some sort of protocol that they had failed to mention during prep. Now my nostrils itched something fierce, yet I couldn't communicate my discomfort, which may be the most frustrating feeling on the planet, if you think about it. I began to store small amounts of oxygen into my lungs and force light puffs of carbon dioxide through my nostrils in a lame attempt to relieve the annoyance. It didn't work. In a far more forceful approach, I tried to free my arms from the bolts and straps that presumably were holding them tight to my sides. Again, no dice.

The next time that the lady came over to analyze me, I made sure to remain awake. She smiled while I began a desperate campaign of awkward signing. My eyes remained focused on her and began looking down, then up again, in repetitive motions, trying to get her to pick up on the signal. She raised her hands to my face as if to understand the instructions that I was miming. Then I watched her slowly move a tube from my nose, and I felt an immediate sense of relief. My eye gestures surely explained the act of gratitude as she adjusted the tube accordingly. At this point, it was clear that negligible consciousness was now setting in as the sleep-induced concoction they had administered began to wane.

It becomes a bit frightening as the senses begin to fire back to a permanently "on position," which is what happened over the course of a couple hours after the surgery was finished. The senses of time, sight, speech, and smell get restored gradually. It's like the feeling of walking out of a casino at seven thirty in the morning after a blackjack bender. It takes those thirty seconds to a minute when you do your best to piece together the evening's events—that moment when you feel pathetically sleep deprived, painfully hung over, bizarrely hungry, and shamefully down in chip count, because you simply insisted on playing for just an hour more. That's the pit feeling of waking up after surgery. Eventually, all senses begin to wake up to the point that you start putting the timeline together. However, everything that occurred in between is unknown. Your voice starts to reestablish word as well as sentence structure. When staff would come to my side to check on me, I could make out their words, then respond in a weak and broken-up tone. Someone asked me if I knew where I was. My goddamn hands were still restrained to my sides and I demanded explanation as to why they were swaddled in this manner. Even my legs had a pins-and-needles sensation like they were asleep, which grew extremely agitating, as I lay there motionless in recovery.

Finally, at some moment, I saw him coming toward me from the right-hand side. It was Berman. To my recollection, he walked over and gave me the once-over and patted my leg before departing from my bedside. I truly don't think he said a word. I was still so out of it that it probably wouldn't have mattered anyway, but good grief, man. A simple "Hey, bud, how are you feeling?" would have been a nice gesture on his behalf after busting open my skull. There was no update, no action plan, and no positive words affirming what had taken place two hours before. I didn't think much of it and then he was gone.

At some point, I came to yet again in that recovery area to find my family hovering over me in a most curious fashion. I recognized everyone immediately and instinctively intended to take Christy's hand in a mutual effort of comfort, but with no success. They still had me bolted down to the board. Now, I was aware of my surroundings enough to explain my discomfort in soft-voiced broken sentences. "Please tell them to free my arms up," I pleaded in a meek tone. Christy carefully lowered the blanket exposing my arms, which were saturated with tubes and intravenous lines, as well as foreign instrument cables that hung down from all directions. My arms were completely numb and did not move. My initial assumption was incorrect. I was not affixed to the bed. We would ask the nurse about the discomfort upon her next visit. This point allowed for a small sigh of relief by all. Dr. Berman had in fact gone out to the waiting area to debrief my squad before joining me in the recovery unit. The surgeon had explained that all had gone according to plan. The mass had been successfully drained, then removed, and a portion of the cyst would be taken to the nearby lab where they would perform a biopsy. Berman also informed them that there was no detection of a "bleed," which meant that no apparent trauma was sustained during the course of the procedure. This was obviously an added statement of a successful overall outcome. And though I felt like complete dog shit, a festive vibe started to take shape in that recovery area.

A couple of other post-surgery patients were also in this area where they were being reunited with their loved ones and friends. The staff checked on us often and we did inquire about the numbness as well as the immobility in both my arms and legs. We were informed that the feeling of numbness was indeed a typical post-surgery symptom, especially when a right-side temporal procedure was performed. The tingling sensation would likely subside within several hours, we were told. I distinctly remember a guy beside me who'd had a similar sort of operation. He was in close proximity, and though I had limited neck agility, his resting station was in view to my left. This guy was a real pistol in personality, I tell ya, probably around fifty years old. He was up and pacing about to the fullest extent that the wires and tubes would allow, likely without any permission to do so by credentialed staff. My family was conversing with a couple of his guests as well. He had a huge gauze wrap on his head and had been confined to one of these exquisite operating beds as well, loaded up with multiple monitors attached to his body that most likely were similar in function to mine. This gave clear evidence that the he also had gone through a large medical undertaking that morning. Yet his overall demeanor was far more chipper and upbeat than mine. He was on the prowl, inquiring about having a ham and cheese sandwich spread delivered to his bedside in short order. This guy was either a pain tolerance powerhouse or had been through this sort of drill before.

Let's just say that on this day of surgery, I was not going to rebound like my neighbor. This sort of frustrated me. Listen, I knew that there was going to be a recovery time denominator in the equation. From what I gathered from those around me, we'd had a procedure that was quite similar in nature (then again, I could be quite wrong). This character was in much better shape than I was. Perhaps he had a better reaction to the anesthesia or possibly his operation was less invasive than mine in some way. The point being, if I had rebounded as he was doing, I would have chalked the day up as a success. A pattern of recovery would unfold and I would be back to my day-to-day in no time.

At some point hours later (which felt like an absolute eternity), I was taken to the ICU for observation. My bones felt extremely weak. Both my arms and legs remained limp and debilitated. The machines continued to ring out in all directions. The machine at the bottom of the bed, which fired every couple of minutes, was connected to my ankles. They had explained that they use this device to monitor blood pressure in the legs to prevent blood clots from forming. Each ankle was fitted into a plastic sleeve that looked like a floatie that you put on a child's arms when learning to swim. The pain was excruciating on my legs as the plastic sacs filled then released approximately sixty seconds later. The noise in itself was extremely rattling, especially while trying to sleep.

My family and staff got me comfortable in my new room on my new floor. I wanted to ask Berman about when this unresponsive limb condition would pass. A nurse came in to check on me, so I inquired. She said at this hour he likely wouldn't be in to follow up until tomorrow. She gave me a tucking in of sorts and I had no problem at all drifting off for a long night of rest and repair.

The staff woke me early on day one after surgery. Honestly, I didn't understand why. The whole game plan was for me to get plenty of rest and now they were waking me up at 7:00 A.M.? I was being fed intravenously and had no appetite. They had catheted me at some point the day before, so using the bathroom was not an issue. A morphine drip was administered after the drugs wore off from yesterday's procedure, so there was no pain management issue either. So, what was going on around here? My head throbbed something awful and my brain was extremely groggy as I began to piece together the prior day's events. My arms were still asleep. My legs felt the same tingle. Even my eyesight felt extremely unbalanced and hazy. I've never experienced vertigo sickness (thank heavens), but my eyes couldn't adjust to simple items or people's faces. The result was a feeling of brief dizziness and confusion. Upon the nurse's arrival, I reported these basic findings and was told that the doctor would be in at some point to give me a follow-up. Berman had prescribed a CT scan to be run, which now explained the early wake-up call. They needed to see if they in fact got what they were going in for.

Back upstairs, the wait for the doctor began. As family filed in to my room for the day's visit, I was becoming even more restless about this whole arms and legs situation. The pressure in my head became agonizing. At some point, I finally caught a glimpse of myself in a mirror. The reflection was something dreadful in nature. It was surreal how swollen my face had become in twenty-four hours. My eyes looked like I'd been slugged in the back of the head with a baseball bat. A thick white bandage traveled from the middle of my eyebrow all the way up to form sort of a skullcap. This was exactly what the chipper guy resting beside me in recovery had on. You could just make out where the staples began above my right eye. A thicker layer of bandage was applied to the right front, which obviously was where they'd opened up the bone in my skull. You could see a thick brown paste at the start of the abrasion, which I later learned was applied to prevent infection while containing a bonding adhesive to seal the wound. Staring at this practically unrecognizable face, I attempted to gesture myself with a fake smile. I noticed immediately that the muscles on the left side of my mouth weren't responding. There was a noticeable droop, which I chose to blow off in the moment. Putting this all into perspective as I analyzed my current state, a particular thought overwhelmed me. What Berman had described to us was understated. This was by no means a typical procedure. This was indeed a massive, invasive operation.

"Where the hell is this son of a bitch?" That was the question on all of our minds as early evening set in. Without trying to sound agitated, we asked nurses and aides on multiple occasions when Berman would be in to give us the latest updates and lab results. We each started to form our own lists of inquiries as we waited for the debriefing. The nurses who cared for me on that ICU floor remained positive and calm, assuring us that we would have answers soon as to why my post-surgery condition was not improving. We all had a hunch that the staff was not permitted to provide us with updates. The post-surgery evening turned to night with no sign that Berman would check in as promised. He never showed that evening.

But do you know who did show up? Doug and Leon came in for a post-operation assessment. If anyone could cheer me up, it was these two! And it shifted my attitude completely. I was so excited to see them that I could barely see straight—both figuratively and literally! They were obviously very concerned as Christy and my mom had filled them in on the whole situation. They didn't grasp the reasoning of why the doctor hadn't shown on this particularly crucial day either. The sight of my condition alone was enough to signal some sort of warning siren of sorts. My comprehension was very much on point, but my speech was considerably weakened. They kept their concern to themselves, though, as the typical banter and office chatter filled the room. "Fret not, fellas," I muttered. "I'll be in top shape and back in no time at all!" "We know you will," they both confirmed. The mood remained light yet energetic, which was precisely how the three of us collaborated on a daily basis. They made me feel as though I was still plugged in on the work front. We all laughed and talked shop, keeping the mood as positive as could be expected given the circumstances.

Each time a professional would come into the room, Leon would refer to them by the name of "Doctor." Every nurse, technician, person who brought up an evening snack, blood pressure and temperature-taking attendant, janitor, and intravenous bag level checker got fed the same label. It was an absolute circus, they all must have thought. I laughed like a hyena each and every time. Perhaps it's one of those "you had to be there to appreciate it moments," but Leon's delivery was spot on that evening. (I'm cracking up as I type this just thinking about it.) Just seeing those two inspired me to be patient as we figured this all out. My mood was grateful that evening, surrounded by all of my friends and loved ones. Even though we didn't have the answers we were in search of, everything would get ironed out in short order. Tomorrow would be a new day!

You know that feeling when you haven't exercised a certain set of muscles in a while, so you figure they need a thorough workout? The next day, it doesn't hurt much, but the day after that you feel as though you got hit by a truck. That is precisely how I felt on February 24, 2006, which was two days after my surgery. That was the morning that the physical pain officially set in. Every muscle in my body ached something awful. Each lifeless limb cramped as if torqued by a vice grip. My head throbbed from the line of incision to the back of my brain stem. The line from "He's Gone" by the Grateful Dead came to mind: "I'll steal your face right off your head." And that's exactly how I felt—simply "gone." "How does it hurt to blink?" I thought. "Furthermore, how can you possibly get through a particular day without blinking?" There wasn't enough morphine or plush pillows on this floor to ease the symptoms that I felt once I woke up. A nurse did increase my morphine drip as I do recall. You could just see the pain in my swollen face. I looked like shit and felt far worse. "Where's this goddamn doctor?" I slurred.

On day three of still no professional update on my condition to this point, a nurse finally informed me that a doctor was on the floor and would be in to see me shortly. "Listen, that's all fine and good, but I need Berman in here immediately to tell me what's going on. Look at me! I can't get out of bed!" Phone calls were made to get my family over here at once. Now three days past surgery, the laundry list of questions was growing by the hour. We all needed to get some understanding and direction on what the next steps looked like. The one positive leading up to this point was that my right arm was slowly waking up. My fingers fired and the ability to pivot my elbow was restored. I was permitted to order breakfast, giving me the first solid nutrients that I'd been able to ingest since Tuesday. When the breakfast was served, the entire task of simply positioning myself to eat was an ordeal. You have to keep in mind that I held a pretty fit frame at the time, which was a good thing until the staff had to reposition

175 pounds of dead weight just to get a feeding tray in front of me. The entire process took two assistants to prop me up with pillows in order to complete the task. Just the simple act of clinching my fork was extremely difficult. The feeling of cold metal from the spoon felt like nails being jabbed into my fingers. The exercise of eating was too much for me to handle, and a nurse was summoned to assist me. So now I was coming to realize that not only was my body partially paralyzed, but also my sensory receptors were not firing correctly. Each and every major body shift brought upon an excruciating level of pain. I felt awful making the staff work that hard just to tend to my needs. I could tell by the look in their eyes that they felt bad for my current situation. They were all uplifting and put a positive spin on an extremely frustrating set of circumstances.

My family came into my room some hours later, and amazingly, the doctor followed behind moments thereafter. This was not Dr. Berman as we were promised but a general practitioner of sorts who was making his rounds on the ICU. Collaboratively, we weren't sure whether to feel misled or relieved upon his arrival. This was to be one of the very first doctors to analyze my current state of affairs and give us all some much-needed feedback. As the doctor began his assessment, questions tumbled out of the mouths of all five of us. His demeanor was very professional, yet he rapidly appeared over-whelmed by our onslaught. The intent was not to blame him for the lack of follow-up but rather to point out the obvious. "Something is clearly wrong with Jonathan's recovery from what we were told going into his surgery. We need basic questions answered now if his doctor is not on-site!" This was the first blanket statement voiced by my mother, not to state the obvious or anything. This poor guy knew within two minutes of this particular room visit that he was going to be forced to lie on multiple hand grenades through no fault of his own. He began checking my vitals as the volleys continued from all directions of the room. My intuition told me that he knew that some-thing was way off as a result of the surgery. He knew that something was seriously wrong. The doctor began to choose his wording very carefully. His observations were presented extremely broadly from his area of expertise. He clearly wanted out of that room while giving us as little explanation of my status as humanly possible.

The entire visit took less than eight minutes. He came up with some bullshit line that the surgeon's notes from Wednesday's operation provided a much clearer explanation as to why I wasn't responding accordingly. "Great," I exclaimed in frustration. "When am I going to see the goddamn doctor as promised?" He had no answer, nor did anyone else in this forsaken place! Someone in the room reversed the interrogation. "Listen, it is currently late Friday morning. Should we assume that Berman is not going to pay us a three-day-overdue visit over the course of this weekend?" The doctor played it safe with the "I know not what the doctor's weekend schedule looks like" line. "Well, then, can you reach out to him on our behalf to explain the situation?" someone blared out. "I will see what I can do to make contact," assured the doctor. Was a rebuttal given? A hunch tells me that very little effort was put into fulfilling this request. And then he was gone.

We all looked at one another, confused, concerned, and pissed off by what had just transpired. Personally, it all made sense to me. I was no patient of this guy. Furthermore, he wouldn't be held responsible for giving us his prognosis without fully understanding the circumstances. But something was dreadfully wrong here. Half of my body wasn't working for whatever reason and Berman had disappeared. My mother was furious, Christy was livid, and I was frantic.

A few hours later, I was informed that a physical therapist was coming in to do an evaluation on me. We had no idea if this was typical protocol on the unit or if the doctor from earlier had arranged the consultation. A real nice guy came to my room shortly thereafter and told me that he wanted to conduct a series of tests. I did my best to fill him in on the events of the last few days. Just thinking about the order in which the days fell made me very tired. He asked me to perform several movements with my right arm, wrist, and fingers. He noticed that the muscles were firing but were still weak. This was to be expected considering the location of the incision placement just above the right temporal lobe. He moved to my left arm. Nothing. No movement whatsoever. I did have some sensation when it came to touch, but nothing fired. He told me to focus and concentrate on moving my fingers. They remained locked in a clenched fist as if someone had replaced the tendons with concrete. Every muscle was extremely tight, almost to a locked position with very little range of motion.

The therapist then focused on my legs. I did notice some control of my right leg, although the tingly feeling was dominant. I distinctly remember feeling a sensation as he manipulated the limb. But switching to the left, I felt nothing at all. It might as well have been detached for all I could tell. All my joints felt as if they'd rusted together with no give due to long periods of weather exposure. It was so frustrating even to describe to this professional. It was as if a circuit breaker had flipped and refused to switch back to the On position. My right leg checked out as functional for the most part with only sensation issues. My left leg was completely unresponsive. Suddenly, as he actively yet cautiously moved the limb, I shrieked in pain and my left leg returned to a neutral position. He then tried to calibrate a benchmark for range of motion, but there was scarcely any movement to report. My foot dangled from the side of the bed, lifeless. Muscles refused to fire from my hip to my toes. He took notes rigorously. My head and neck movements checked out well except for my mouth movements, which were still impacted on the left side.

We began to talk once his assessment was concluded. "They can't tell us much because the doctor who performed the surgery hasn't been by to assess my situation yet. We're just looking for some answers here," I said. "Sometimes these muscles will begin to refire after a few days just like your right side has begun to do," he explained. "Other times they need assistance waking up and that's what we help you with in PT. Other times, the muscles refuse to respond due to the break in signal between the brain and muscle. We find ways to work around that as well." "So, you can tell that something is not right with my situation, correct?" I asked. "Yes," he said. "But it is way too early for me to tell where you're at in all of this. It's going to take time." "I'll do whatever it takes to get back to work and play my guitars." I was confident in my words. "That's a great attitude to have!" he assured me.

I was instructed to rest up through the weekend and we would likely start therapy at the beginning of next week. He was a good dude and I was pretty excited that this guy at least gave it to me straight while explaining what the next steps were. By that evening, there was still no sign of the doctor (nor would there be through the weekend, I kept reminding myself). However, on a positive, my sales reps showed up for a while to talk shop, following up from the past week. Regardless of my current situation, they knew it was important to keep me in the know in sort of a roundtable Friday-morning-meeting fashion. Greg, Bobby, Kevin, and Mike knew this would cheer me up. The sheer sight of me would likely shake them a touch. A week ago, I was the guy staying a few days in the hospital making sure that everything checked out after the accident. Now, well, this! Regardless, that hour and then some was grand. We talked business for a few, then reminisced about the shenanigans of our Vegas trip from just a few weeks earlier. The atmosphere felt rather surreal in the moment reflecting back. Regardless, fear not, fellas! I would be back at the office ripping around full tilt in no time, I insisted to my troops. We laughed and carried on just as if it were another Friday after work happy hour. We all made the best out of the situation at hand.

Throughout the weekend, several of my staff, office employees, even neighbors dropped by to say hello as word of the surgery spread. It was a great feeling to see everyone. Visitation hours made time speed up while lying in a semi-paralyzed state of being while jailed to a hospital bed. The only options of entertainment get reduced to eating, sleeping, watching weekend television, and visitation. However, despite the circumstances, I did my best to remain in good spirits even though we were all frustrated. Friday's talk with the physical therapist gave me the positive professional insight that I was looking for. Just as with my right arm, the connection between my brain and limbs simply needed a little more time to wake back up. They had to! It only made sense! Berman was not going to show up this weekend. That was made perfectly clear.

The weekend was going to have to ride itself out. The comparison between pre-surgery weekend versus post-surgery weekend became quite obvious. Last weekend I was chewing at the bit to be discharged and get the hell out of here. For post-surgery weekend, I was sick. I mean, truly, truly sick. I needed to be here, and I knew it. When you don't want to be somewhere, like a hospital, the time drags, but when you know in the back of your mind that you indeed need to be in said place, you feel far more appreciative of your surroundings.

The weekend pressed ahead with a great deal of anticipation. Several visitors poured in and out as I was beginning to feel quite restless. By this point, I had been confined to a bed for nearly ninety-six hours straight. And getting me out of bed wasn't even an option. I hadn't been cleared by the doctor (Berman or otherwise) to do so. A shower would have been fabulous but was also out of the question because my headdress (far from a masculine description for gauze wrap that covers the staples) was not permitted to be exposed to moisture. So, the harsh reality here was that, yes, folks, sponge baths and bedpans were needed to get the job done for now.

Monday, February 27, marked my tenth day in the Robert Wood Johnson Hospital. Just like the Monday before, the normal buzz of the unit was back to a full cadence in the morning. My breakfast was delivered, and nurses followed in to raise me in to somewhat of an elevated dining posture after sliding my portable eating desk flush against my chest. Also like the mornings prior, my head hurt something awful. The staff was trying to slowly wean me off of the morphine drip by reducing the flow during the night. The result was a skull-thumping headache as my eyes adjusted to the lighting and my body sensitivity inputs were becoming antiquated in this new skin.

Unlike the previous mornings, the thought didn't even come across my mind to ask if "my" doctor was coming in to check on me today. By this point, Christy, my mother, Doug, and Leon had planted the seeds that if we didn't hear from my brain surgeon today, steps for patient neglect were going to be acted upon. Leon sought legal counsel through a family member who did agree upon explanation of the scenario that some sort of distinguished follow-up was certainly lacking here. The doctor who'd dropped in on Friday did at least have the courtesy to stop by again today. He went through with his normal routine and did speak up to say that he had left multiple messages with Berman's office that his attention to the matter was requested immediately. Strangely, I didn't believe him in the least on Friday, but his words resonated today. So, once again, we all waited for the better half of the day. At some point that afternoon, there was confirmation that he was coming in to discuss operation specifics. It seemed to me that multiple staff members were relieved by this news as well. There are only so many times within a given day where five people are asking the same question over and over again as to the whereabouts of this clown.

Early that evening, Old Berman finally showed up—completely expressionless, just as he had been days ago when we all first met.

What do you say in a moment like this? You can't just blurt out, "Hey, cowboy, where the fuck have you been?" in utter frustration. He walked in with his binders and such, then turned to acknowledge the room as if he were about to plagiarize Churchill's "We Shall Fight on the Beaches" speech. He surely could see in our eyes what was on our minds as he tried to read his audience before delivering the results of the CT scan. "I want to apologize for the delay in response," he started in a mumble. "I was on holiday over the past few days."

So, let's stop right here for a second. You were on vacation, you say? Well, all right, I get that. A long weekend getaway, perhaps. But aren't there backup procedures in place for this?

I don't remember who fired the first missile (Christy or my mother, if I were to guess). "In our post-surgery debriefing, you pointed out that you detected no evidence of 'brain bleed,' which to our understanding meant that everything went according to plan. Well, look at his condition now! Is this your definition of 'according to plan,' Doctor?" Berman then approached me from the left side of the bed. And began a physical examination of his own, which was far less extensive than the physical therapist's. He focused on my arm first. He observed my clenched fist, which remained so tight that the fingers snapped back into a locked fist immediately after extending to a neutral position. He told me to smile and could see the facial droop in my eye and on my mouth. My leg was then analyzed. There was no movement from hip to toes. Then it was time for him to proceed to the other side of the bed. The doctor admired his staple job that ran from above my right eye and ended in a site that I was not aware of because of the gauze wrapping covering the wound. He carefully inspected the now bonded crevice with his fingers. That pressure was felt above my eye socket, and the light compressing made me wince a little, so he stopped.

Our audience watched intently. Berman then slowly migrated over to the images on the reader board and sort of glanced over them as if he hadn't seen them before. One feature was very striking, which I noticed right off the bat, as he analyzed the before and the after images. There was an enormous black crater/cavity/abyss in the middle right on my skull. He explained where he went in, and there was now no doubt that what he had gone in to retrieve was gone. An overwhelming black void from the top of my brain was all that remained. The sight was very impressive to view in real time. The doctor then spoke up. "There is good news to report and not so good news to report. The positive is that the biopsy culture came back clean." This meant that the mass turned out to be benign. My mom and I made eye contact, and slight smiles of relief were exchanged. "The other side of the coin," he explained, "is that some sort of CVA episode has taken place and we should schedule a follow-up MRI immediately for review of the impacted region."

This is what I got out of those five minutes of data explained by a person who may be the most pathetically weak communicator

I've ever encountered: "The findings were that there was no sign of cancer detected. That's great!" You then follow that remark up with (presumably) a medical acronym in which no one in the room except for the presenter knows anything about. Shall we try this approach, "Senior Doctor"? "What the fuck is going on with the left side of my body anyway?"

He continued on, "Upon release from ICU and pending the results of testing from the MRI, we will make specific arrangements to transport Jonathan to a rehabilitation facility, which will complement his medical needs going forward." Again, in my head I'm thinking, "Why the hell are you sending me to another hospital? I need to get back to work! You told me that in a couple weeks that you would clear me, and all would be well!" My mood became noticeably grim. A wave of scared discomfort grew in the pit of my stomach. The message delivered was that I was truly in deep trouble physically and I didn't understand why this bastard couldn't explain to a ten-year-old how to make a peanut butter and jelly sandwich, yet they had given him an advanced degree in how to split people's heads open to conduct brain surgery. "This is completely fucking absurd!" I thought. The defense mechanism, in what was left of my brain, kicked in. I shut down completely, like when my father would scold me to release his stress rather than correct the action. This low-level simpleton couldn't even communicate effectively as to what the degree of his mistake had been during some point during the operation. Furthermore, he backed off after his official opinion was addressed to the room. There was neither a rally speech nor an aggressive plan of action devised. That feeling was heartbreaking. I was utterly demoralized in that moment; I will never forget it.

My family raised additional concerns. Berman responded with a weary, weak demeanor as if he were giving a eulogy at a funeral rather than consulting with his damaged patient. He informed us that he would return tomorrow to review the results of the MRI.

The one positive to report from the prior evening's meeting of the minds was that Berman did clear me for bed release. This meant that with the help and strength of multiple professionals, they were allowed to transfer me from my bed into a chair or wheelchair. The task was brutally challenging on both sides of the fence. The pain felt something awful as my sensory signals were extremely receptive to touch. For the staff, it meant lifting my 175 pounds of dead weight with wires and tubes connected all over. Yet, the permission did serve as my first sense of independence. This would also serve as a useful grant of access for the next morning as the MRI runners were able to transport me down to the tube without the bulky operation bed getting in the way. Three members of that team hoisted me from chair to plank, which was terribly uncomfortable at the time, yet I knew these results were going to be extremely important in diagnosing my condition. They settled me in, and the table then drifted back into the sphere where the racket of clangs, knocks, clunks, and buzzes did not affect that tight environment that I was becoming increasingly familiar with.

Surprisingly, Berman was on point once the results came through late that afternoon. Personally, I didn't want to have anything to do with the bastard but did want to know the results of the MRI. My mom, Christy, and I were waiting for him. He walked in and was content to see me sitting upright in a chair opposite from my bed. I was simply ecstatic to be out of bed even for a half hour or so at a clip before exhaustion set in. He moped into the room, same as the times before. What kept running through my brain was, "Where the hell did this hack go on vacation?" He looked like he'd be miserable on just about any landmark on the planet. Perhaps he had some swanky beach house on the Jersey Shore. (But that made no sense going into March. It was freezing down there at this time of year.) Perhaps the gulf coast of Florida where he had to take his snot-nosed grandkids once a year. Or maybe he was on a chess retreat in Vermont. The possibilities of ridiculous destinations were endless. He again approached me and started the same game of checking and testing my limbs. "I've got news for you, pal—no change to speak of!" I thought, shrieking inside.

After approximately five minutes of contorting my paralyzed limbs, he stood up from his squatting position to address us. "Though I did not see any type of 'bleed' during the surgery, I did notice an extremely small abrasion on the back of Jonathan's thalamus, which may be blocking the signals from the right side of the brain to the left side. This may be the result of a specific tool that was placed on the back of his head during the operation. The tool may have nicked a blood vessel at some point during the procedure, which may have resulted in weakness on the left side. Every CVA"—there was that word again—"is different in severity as well as recovery," he stated. He then put an image onto the now lit-up reading board. An image of the very back of my head was in view. With a thin pen, which he pulled out of his examination coat, he pointed to a speck on the image that was no longer than an eyelash and no thicker than a fruit fly. "This is what I believe is causing the paralysis in this case." We all looked at each other, then back at Berman. "You may make a full recovery and you may not. My advice at this point is to transfer you to a rehabilitation hospital where the staff is trained in recovery from this sort of traumatic brain injury."

I looked at the diagram on the screen and then back at him. "So, what you are telling us here is that this almost non-visible wound somehow blew out the left side of my body?"

"That is my educated guess at this point," he said in a low voice. "This outcome is very rare but does occur in some cases during invasive procedures such as this."

Author's Note:

Cerebrovascular accident (CVA) is the medical term for a stroke. A stroke is when blood flow to a part of your brain is stopped either by a blockage or the rupture of a blood vessel. There are important signs of a stroke that you should be aware of and watch out for.

* * *

"And just to be clear, I am twenty-eight years old and have had a stroke? Well, what the hell does that mean?" I screeched. "Kids in high school have heat strokes because of excess heat exposure during games and practices"—attempting to prove my knowledge on the subject.

"Strokes and brain injury of this magnitude come in all shapes and sizes," he explained. "Well, when can I go back to work?" I asked, panic-stricken. "I don't know," he said lowly. At that moment, the floor was all that I chose to gaze at. I didn't care to see anyone or their expressions. As I saw it, this meeting was over. I have no memory as to the events that immediately followed. Perhaps they all reconvened in the hall to discuss next steps while I processed the news. The pressure in the room felt overpowering. Perhaps they left me in silence to collect my thoughts.

Eventually, they all began to filter back into the room. Each held onto a positive demeanor, but I wasn't buying into any of the bullshit. Christy and the doctor were the last to enter, their presence like an order to call the room back to order. Berman's approach when he started back up was lax and effortless as he began to mumble his opinions and findings yet again. The interpretation became clear in those moments—that *he* was responsible for this CVA incident he spoke of. "I am going to release Jonathan from ICU tomorrow morning and he will be transported to JFK Johnson Rehabilitation Institute in Edison, New Jersey, which is located roughly fifteen minutes from here. There, he will receive the care to get him back to strength while monitoring his recovery. We will reconvene in my office upon his discharge to assess his progress when the time comes."

"Well, how long do you think they're going to keep me in there for?" I inquired. "We have no way of determining a time frame until professional evaluations are conducted," he explained. He then approached me and I fired on him a glare of self-confidence deep from within. He bent over slightly and patted me twice on the thigh. "They'll get you all fixed up over there," he stated through his old, weak smile. He then exited the room. I suppose I would have shrugged my shoulders and said "Oh well" to break the tension of the room, but I couldn't lift my shoulders with my short-circuited muscles. Muscles that simply refused to budge due to reasons in which I did not understand. Furthermore, reasons that were completely out of my control. They brought me into this hospital initially to monitor some bumps and bruises due to a vehicle accident. Now, I would be leaving this place in the morning with a far more acute situation on my plate.

Speaking of "plate in the morning," the morning of the release from Robert Wood Johnson, I ate like a horse in appreciation of the kitchen staff that kept me nourished during my stay with them. I have eaten hospital food at multiple facilities throughout these intervening years, and Robert Wood Johnson's "made to order" approach was a top-shelf experience despite a rather grave set of circumstances.

The nurses and technicians made me aware bright and early that this day of discharge and transfer would be very busy as well as exhausting. IV lines were unscrewed from my arms while monitoring devices were switched off and cords were disconnected from my chest and abdomen. As I recall, the process felt absurdly freeing. Next, a team of three came in the room to explain details of how the transfer was going to be carried out. Christy and my mom had packed up my belongings the night before, figuring that they would just come to the new facility once I got situated over there. So I started to get my affairs in order by saying goodbyes and words of thanks to all of the staff members who'd helped me to this point. They all commented on my positive attitude in one way or another, regardless of where this journey was to lead me in the future. The only disappointment was that I wanted to share my gratitude to those on the previous floor as well. I wanted them to know what happened and where I was off to next to get better. One staff member assured me that the news of my surgery had spread. Yet, who knows if she was being honest or simply wanted to make me feel better with a small white lie? Regardless, I realized that I was only one of likely thousands of patients the staff meets each year. Every patient's journey differs in some capacity. Not every professional is going to remember every admitted patient on a given floor. Even though I certainly wish that were the case, it becomes simply unfeasible.

The transport squad came up to get me just before noon. Three upbeat fellas who were cracking jokes and gawking at female employees is what I remember most as they moved me onto some sort of transportation gurney. These guys whisked me out of the room and off the floor in such a way that they must have been late for their lunch break or perhaps jonesing for a midday smoke. I hardly had a moment to say my goodbyes to everyone at the nurses' station as they whisked me by for the final time. At the elevator, while waiting for our floor to ring out, one of the guys looked at me professionally and said, "Man, what happened to your head?" Now inside the elevator, I entertained them with a summed-up account of what had brought me here. They all gave me positive words of encouragement and strength. The elevator door slid open and again they briskly maneuvered the halls as if a competition was underway to see how fast they could load me up and sweep me out of the joint.

Finally, we approached a set of automated doors that led to an approach to the parking garage. A bitter cold splash of air hit my face with a brutal force at the exit point of the building. The sudden pain was overwhelming. My facial sensory receptors were still extremely delicate and the gusting air forced my tear ducts to erupt; involuntary, tears streamed down my face within seconds. The level of pain was brutal, yet I threw on my best poker face as we raced across the garage. Keep in mind that this was the first time that fresh air had entered my lungs in two weeks. As much as I wanted to embrace the moment, my left side shook something fierce as I could tell it was attempting to fight off the cold sensation that was now rattling my bones. We approached a van that looked like some sort of ambulance hybrid without all the medical bells and whistles. As for the amount of time that had elapsed between leaving the building to the doors closing on the van, I have not a clue. What I can tell you is that it felt like an eternity. They loaded me in with full understanding of the pain that I had just experienced. I was informed that this shuttle ride might be bumpy. I realized within moments what he was talking about as we set off for the garage exit. This van drove like a carnival amusement ride without shocks or power steering. My head felt the effect of every bump. Each striking blow hit harder than the next. As we pulled out onto the local streets, then the highway, I winced every few seconds as my head would slightly recoil off the stretcher. Every pothole, acceleration, and brake maneuver got absorbed through my body over the course of a fifteen-minute ride, which felt like an hour. Destination: JFK rehabilitation hospital.

12

EVERY DAY IS
EXACTLY THE SAME

he transfer crew delivered me to JFK Rehabilitation in the same
fashion as they had gathered me from Robert Wood Johnson
approximately an hour earlier. The facility doors slid open and
they whisked me right past the admissions desk as if they owned the
joint. The destination for my transfer was to take place on the third
floor, they told me. Upon arrival at level three, I took notice of the
signage above. In big black letters over yet another set of electronic
doors, it read "Intensive Care Unit" (ICU) to the right and "Traumatic
Brain Injury" (TBI) to the left. Common sense told me that they'd
likely admit me to the ICU for observation for a night or two based
on my condition, then figure out what to do with me. Rather, the guys
pulled an audible, making a left bank toward the TBI wing without

saying a word. I was baffled in this moment and now most interested in hearing the explanation of the selected wing.

We were met by an extremely friendly staff out front of the nurses' station. The atmosphere was lively and upbeat. Smiling faces greeted me one by one as they analyzed my particulars. The three gentlemen who gave me the lift over were excused and I thanked them for their etiquette in transport. There in that corridor, I waited patiently for further instructions to be carried out. As my ears adjusted, the same sounds of meters and monitors and gauges rang out from all angles of the wing. The warm air within had settled the unnerving pain on my left side. The throbbing pain that picked up momentum in my head was a different situation altogether. The combination of the ride over and my eyes still not being able to focus properly gave me a head thumping of horrendous magnitude. I could feel my pulse underneath the headdress on the incision. In the couple hours that they had disconnected the morphine drip, the effects were felt, unmissable. A pain from within grew terribly sharp. I felt semi-nauseous, yet more than anything a wave of exhaustion passed over like no other.

Several minutes or hours went by. Again I analyzed my surroundings carefully. Sometime later, a nurse came to my bedside. She began asking me a series of questions that I knew all too well by this point. She began, "Do you know where you are? Do you know why you're here? Do you know how you got here?" In the typical protocol, the questions were answered to the best of my knowledge. After the interrogation, I expressed my concern about my aching head. The woman told me that a doctor would be in to evaluate me shortly. "Yeah? I've heard that line before," I thought to myself.

Sometime later, Christy and my mom showed up to check out my new digs on the floor. Naturally, I was very relieved to see them both, but I could tell in their eyes that the emotional strain was real. Especially for Christy. She looked as if she hadn't slept in days, and likely she hadn't. She was doing her best to balance her work responsibilities while taking care of the countless tasks, phone calls, and bedside meetings revolving around my day-to-day condition. The massive load thrust upon her shoulders was excessive. And I could read between the lines in her tone that these recent blindsiding events were not what she'd signed up for when we said our nuptials a mere six months earlier.

They got me adjusted properly as they were now becoming accustomed to positioning me accordingly for mealtimes and visitors. The details of my transfer were softly explained and I told them about the severe pain in my head. To this point, my level of pain tolerance was fairly strong, given the circumstances. Yet now, off of powerful sedatives, the ache set in something awful. The nurse had informed me earlier that the doctor would likely prescribe a medication that would dull the pain. But when would that be? The thumping ebbed and flowed more intensely as each hour passed. Finally, shortly before evening set in, the doctor arrived at my bedside.

His name was Dr. Urs, an outgoing, dark-haired gentleman who carried himself in an upbeat manner. He had a female assistant with him and they complemented one another nicely. We started with small talk as he observed my condition; then he started performing an overall examination to further assess my current state of affairs. The information on my case provided by nurses at RWJ (I'd assume) aligned with what the three of us were describing as he began a second series of tests on my extremities and face. He was informed of my discomfort as well from the day's earlier events. Once complete, with no sign of improvement over what I had noticed during the past week, he stood up and addressed the room. "First off, the staff and I are going to conduct several more intrusive evaluations starting tomorrow morning. Seeing that tomorrow is a Friday, we will discuss the initial findings and your therapy will begin on Monday morning. I want you to get plenty of rest from now until then. You will need your strength. Also, I will prescribe a pain medication to ease your discomfort." Check, check, and check, I thought as he debriefed his apprentice in front of us.

"I have a question," I stated while he was gathering up his belongings. "Sure, what's up?" he asked. "Why am I in the traumatic brain injury side of the hospital when they told us that all I had was a stroke?" He stopped what he was doing and approached my bed again. The doctor focused on me as if to make certain that I was ready to pay attention to his answer. He started, "Because your stroke was caused as a result of a brain injury that you sustained as a result of the surgery." I didn't like the use of his wording "your stroke" in the least. This wasn't my stroke! Yet, regardless, I continued on, "But the scans revealed a tiny little tear that happened during the surgery. There is nothing traumatic about that."

"That tiny tear has paralyzed the left side of your body because of its location on the back of your brain stem. Now it is our job as well as yours to get you better as quickly as possible." He meant every word of what he said. I nodded in a manner of disbelief. That extremely nervous sensation started to set into my gut again, which didn't help the pulsing that was currently pounding through my head. "Your journey to recovery from this point is not going to be easy, yet we will find a way to help your body recover as best as we can," he finished. The words clung in the room among us all. A feeling of defeat that was not of my doing filled my body. The words began to depress me greatly, yet I chose not to show emotion.

After Doctor Urs and staff left, my dinner was brought in and the three of us arranged me properly. There was precious little chatter amongst us and I ate very little of my dinner that evening. Several minutes later, the nurse arrived with an oral dose of pain medication as well as other prescribed meds. As I thanked her for dropping off the goods, she looked at my dinner tray and smirked as a school-teacher might after catching wind of a disruptive student being caught in the act of mischief. "That's all you're eating this evening?" she inquired. I answered honestly by explaining that my head was hurting something awful and exhaustion was setting in rapidly by this point. Even though it was nice having company by my bedside to help acclimate me to my new surroundings, they could tell that the nurse's assessment from this morning was accurate when she'd pronounced that this day of transfer was going to be draining. Both visitors quickly took the hint that my brain was in need of rest. After evening hugs, kisses, and good nights were exchanged, Christy and Mom left.

My new surroundings felt dark and quiet. All that was to be heard was a distant buzzing sound coming from the nurses' station. The only source of light was from the hallway, and I asked for the door to be left ajar. Within minutes of the painkillers hitting my bloodstream, the physical pains magically drifted off somewhere else. My emotional state became tormented, however, as the words spoken by Dr. Urs played through my head over and over. This accident was in no way my fault—or was it? If a more fitting surgeon would have picked up my case when I first was admitted, or if I would have gotten a second medical opinion before I gave him permission to operate, or If I would have been up front about the episodes that may have caused the accident on Route 18—could this all have been avoided in some way?

For the first time in twelve days, my tear ducts filled and I cried softly. The weight of the situation finally took hold. To this point, my spirits had been upbeat and the outlook on recovery had been positive. However, at this moment, alone in an unfamiliar environment, in an unfamiliar body, I cradled the limp left arm with my semi-functional right. My instinct was to coddle the impacted limb just as a mother would protect her young in that crucial period in the days following birth. The fingers remained clenched into a firm fist and could not be pulled apart. The upper part of my arm rested as limber as a folded sock. And hence, I started to ponder, how could this have happened to me? Why now? When was everything going to wake up? When would they let me go home? How did I have a stroke? Why was my brain injured? These were the questions that raced through my head as I lay there in a state of disbelief. Shorty thereafter, the medication kicked in. My damp eyes and weary mind carried the gravity of cinder blocks as I crashed into a deep slumber.

The next morning, the same familiar buzz filled the halls. Breakfast was served, meds were distributed, and morning bodily functions were extracted accordingly. Upon retrieval of my finished breakfast tray, a nurse came in to the room and began writing an itinerary on the dry erase board positioned on the wall to my left just past the entrance. My eyes still were experiencing difficulty with clarity. They focused just enough to make out the words: "Physical Therapy Eval 10:00, Occupational Therapy Eval 1:00, Speech Pathology Eval 2:00, Dr. Urs consult 3:00." The nurse briskly jotted this on the board in blue marker and in typical womanly penmanship. She informed me that, each day, my schedule would be updated accordingly between therapy sessions and doctor appointments. I nodded, acknowledging the purpose of the board. "Now rest up before your first appointment arrives," she instructed.

On the dot, two young professionals dressed in blue scrubs, one female, the other male, both probably between twenty-five and thirty, entered the room and introduced themselves. They conducted a series of tests focusing on my leg, feet, arms, and head. The evaluation had the feeling of the one conducted at Robert Wood a week prior. After forty-five minutes of information gathering, they said something to the effect of, "We'll see you on Monday," and left the room.

Shortly thereafter, another professional arrived conducting all sorts of physical test on my arms, fingers, and elbows. After lunch, I was subjected to a machine that monitored my speech, sight, and hearing. Some of the evaluations seemed repetitious, yet I figured that there must have been some sort of method to their madness. Christy and Mom arrived shortly before Dr. Urs was to drop in and I recapped all that had happened thus far. Every professional that dropped by was upbeat and personal with me. I immediately liked the environment despite the circumstances that had brought me here. Everyone wanted to know my story to some degree. They empathized with my situation, yet appreciated my high energy level.

When Dr. Urs came into the room, once again with his female counterpart, they began checking my vitals and staples, as done the day before. All of the testing from today came back in the norm of what was to be expected. He made it known to each of us that the staff was looking forward to working with me because of my age and attitude (but honestly, I didn't understand what one had to do with the other). I still was excited that others had pointed out my attitude, for I was very cognizant of the energy that I put off in my new surroundings. The doctor went over a few details of what I was to expect for the next week. "It's going to be five straight days of intense therapy," he explained, reiterating what he'd said yesterday. He approached my bed just as he had the day before, but his tone was a little more relaxed now. "We have three rules here to ensure that you hit your full recovery potential." I shifted myself upright a little, showing that I was indeed paying attention. "You have to get a lot of rest because you will tire quickly. You need to eat regularly so your body sustains energy during your therapy sessions, and speaking of regular, well, you need to be just that, meaning if you get backed up back there, you need to let us know because the effects will bog you down and make you tired." I nodded with each request. "By the way," Urs said, "have you been regular since the surgery?" "Not really," I confessed. "I always have trouble when I'm in foreign environments." "Well, let's keep an eye on it, and if we need to take necessary measures, we will," he instructed. "Also, Doc," I said before they set off to make their rounds to other patients, "is there any chance that I can take an actual shower at some point soon? I mean, these sponge baths just aren't cutting it." He chuckled at the request and told me that he'd see what he could do about that. He did deliver on the request that night.

So, I simply must explain how showering and toileting work when you don't have functioning legs. They have this device that is constructed out of PVC pipe with adaptable wheels, which serves as a makeshift wheelchair complete with grips for steering from the back, as well as a hinged bar that snaps down into place from one armrest to the other a little above the thighs as sort of a lap belt. In the middle, the seat is simply a toilet seat. Somehow, they engineered this contraption so that support is not needed from the back wheels. Therefore, a nurse can simply position the chair above the toilet so that the patient can take care of business. The chair can also assist with showering. Point being, it's not a pretty exercise for anyone involved.

Anyhow, the doctor gave the nurses permission to allow me to shower that evening so long as my head dressing and exposed staples were covered. To say that I was thrilled about a thorough bathing would be an understatement. I waited patiently that evening in anticipation for when the nurses would give me a proper delousing. Finally, a nurse named Wanda came into the room. She hustled to retrieve the showering apparatus on wheels. My facial expression was that of a three-year-old about to gorge on a chocolate cupcake as together we de-robed me, then transferred me from bed to chair. This woman had the strength of an African bush elephant as she transitioned my dead weight onto the chair. Then into the shower we went. Remembering about my skin sensitivity, I asked her to set the water to a lukewarm temperature so that my body would slowly adjust. She maneuvered the chair up, over, then down the ramp into the refreshing strands of warm water. It felt incredible. I would have been content if she would have let me relax in that water for an hour, but the moisture buildup may have compromised my skull wrap so we acted quickly, with her doing a majority of the heavy lifting in washing me.

When we were finished and the water was shut off, my skin sensors reacted accordingly as the now cold feeling of chilled air brushed over me. It felt as if every muscle in my body tightened at once, especially my left arm and leg, which shook uncontrollably. Wanda could tell that the sensation made me nervous as she rapidly toweled the water off. She calmed me by saying that this reaction was quite common and would settle down in time. The feeling of having my limbs shake uncontrollably was one that I was not likely to forget. The sensation of spastic pain hit so hard that all I could think of doing was getting back to bed. Wanda knew that I was extremely uncomfortable, so after a quick toweling off and teeth scrubbing, she whisked me out of the bathroom and into bed. Before this final transfer, she dusted me down with a few shots of baby powder, which, to this day, puzzles me. Perhaps that's some sort of female sleep-well tactic. I need to ask a female nurse about that! She transferred me into bed, and the feeling of the warm sheets settled the spasms down in short order. The task was physically draining. She tidied up the room, then set out to retrieve my nightly medicine: Dilantin (a powerful anticonvulsant) as well as pain medication.

That evening, as I settled in for yet another weekend stay in a hospital, I had a different outlook from the sadness and fear that had racked my brain the previous night. Today had been a good day. The people around me cared about my recovery and goals. A mindset fell into place that whatever this illness or injury was, I had to beat it. The weekend settled in and I was excited to start therapy on Monday.

* * *

The weekend passed quickly with several visitors dropping by to check in on my status. All could tell that I was excited to report that I would be starting therapy on Monday. The nurses also wanted to acclimate me to the gym located at the end of the hall on my floor where, it was explained, a majority of my physical and occupational therapy would be taking place. The room looked like a mid-sized workout room consisting of multiple blue-padded tables that sat a couple of feet off the ground. There were parallel bars, several full-length mirrors, and a five- or six-step wooden staircase with adjustable railings on each side. The room was stocked with all sorts of medicine balls, yoga balls, plastic stretch bands of different shapes and sizes, cones, sports equipment, and devices mounted upon tables, some that looked very complex and others that looked rather primitive in nature. There were several large tables spread out around the perimeter, which were as large as drafting tables yet looked as if they were used for some sort of ongoing craft course. I had the sense that all of these devices and contraptions would become very familiar to me in the near future.

On my first Monday morning of therapy, a nurse came into my room abruptly at seven to assist in dressing me in workout attire for the day's sessions. This nurse was strict in my trying to put my shirt, pants, and sneakers on with only minimal assistance. I fiddled around with my shirt a bit but had no clue as to getting my head and arms through the openings to complete what was now an almost impossible task. I looked at her in confusion and frustration as she instructed me to start with my affected left side, using the right arm to guide the garment around the left arm; then she helped me to position my head through the top, finally snaking my right arm through the opening to complete the task. It took almost three minutes. She looked at me in a stern fashion. "If you are determined to get out of here anytime soon, you are going to have to learn how to compensate until your left side gets stronger. Now then, let's work on your putting your pants on."

The task was despicably challenging as now I had to lift my paralyzed left leg up with my weakened right hand. My core muscles ignited in pain as I tried with all my might to reach the top opening of the pants to my motionless and locked left foot. Bending my kneecap with my right arm seemed to be the only way that this undertaking was even possible so I experimented with a bending manipulation. The nurse then adjusted my body accordingly by the use of bed adjustment control, in such a way that my left leg, then right, could glide properly into the workout bottoms. "We don't have time to address putting your shoes on before your breakfast gets here so we'll save that for another day." Together, we had spent nearly twenty minutes trying to dress and prepare me for the day's events, and already the fatigue started to set into my head something fierce.

Now, I need to point out that perhaps a loose pattern of medical pampering of sorts had set in, but honestly, what was I to do? My limbs didn't function. Tasks such as dressing, feeding, and toileting had all been conducted by medical staff to that point. I mean, that's what they were there for, right? Well, that may have been considered correct until today. Now, the professionals were there to assist, not to do for me. I sensed that the game was going to be much different going forward. And that it was. She told me to lie back and rest for a few minutes before my medicine and breakfast arrived. Fifteen minutes later, I snapped back to alertness as my morning meal was served. The nurse, returning to the room, instructed me to eat as much as I could without her assistance as she began writing a series of events on the whiteboard. My PT was starting in thirty minutes, followed by OT and then speech therapy. I gave myself a mental pep talk as I waited for my first session to begin. "Belt this nonsense out and get back to your normal life," became the rally cry of the campaign.

A young guy named Jonathan came into my room a few minutes later. He immediately introduced himself and shook my weak-gripped right hand. A wave of embarrassment overwhelmed me. "Sorry," I said and my eyes went to the floor. "For what?" "Because the first thing that I teach my salespeople is to give a solid handshake." He got the message. "We'll work on that," he said with a tone of confidence as he transitioned me from bed to wheelchair. We were heading for the gym at the end of the hall while making small talk.

Upon entering the gym, I could feel a buzz and energy in the room. Yet when I saw the look of several patients, I could tell that most weren't as excited as I to be here. Jonathan wheeled me over to the unoccupied mat and transitioned me from the chair. He then prepared to give me an obviously rehearsed spiel, which I was eager to hear. "The goal of physical therapy is to get your muscles firing as close to before as possible. We are going to stretch and exercise your arms and legs. Even if you can't feel movement right now, that's all right. Just try. Imagine that the signal works between your limbs and your brain. Some of the movements are going to be uncomfortable and sometimes painful. You need to let me know of your pain tolerance. You will likely get tired quickly. All you have to do is try. We will make progress every day if you keep a positive mindset." He was regimented and meant every word of it.

And then we began a series of stretches and weight-bearing exercises. It all hurt like hell. Every bend and manipulation felt like shards of glass being precisely driven into my arms and legs. Even my semi-functional right arm had difficulty with weight-bearing exercises. Regardless of the pain, I dug in and fought through the forced movements, which now felt so foreign through my skin. The therapist bent and twisted and pulled muscles to get a gauge of my range of motion in each limb. He remained positive and upbeat as he made assessments about my injury. I did my best to think through the movements in a vain attempt to reconnect to the complex grid of circuits that carried the signal to nerve endings. He could tell that a degree of frustration was setting in. "Just keep trying," he reminded me as he repeated basic motions such as bending my arm from the elbow or leg from the kneecap over and over again. As we powered through several drills, I became inquisitive about my surroundings. The vibe of the room was quite upbeat and fast paced. As I did a quick scan of the space, I couldn't help but notice that, out of fifteen or so patients, I was certainly the youngest of the bunch. My brain became distracted. Between sets of a particular stretching exercise, I found the timing right to ask a few questions. "Did all these people have strokes? Why am I the youngest patient in here? When do you think my left arm is going to wake up, based on what you see?" were the top three out of roughly three thousand inquiries that I wanted addressed off the top of my head.

Jonathan began to address my questions one by one, almost as if he had been anticipating them. "The patients on this floor have a multitude of different brain injuries," he began. "We typically don't see many patients your age up here. Yet, trust me, we like seeing younger people up here—not because they're sick or anything, but because they typically have a reason to try harder to regain what they can from a functionality standpoint." That made sense, I mentally concluded. "As for your recovery, well, every traumatic brain injury is different from the next. Some people make great strides over the first few months and get pretty much back to normal when they leave. Some need several years of healing and therapy to get the slightest functionality back. It all depends on precisely where the injury took place in the brain. The key here is twofold: Studies have shown that the greatest signs of recovery are detected within the first year of injury. Second, age as well as attitude are both very important components when forecasting the greatest level of patient recovery," he concluded. Even though I was in no mood or mind frame to wrap my already wrapped head around all this logic, the explanation did spark some thought.

At the end of the hour, my body ached and my brain was drained. We'd certainly had a positive session, but I barely had the strength to transition back up to my wheelchair to head back to the room. Every muscle that I had used felt sore and fatigued. My eyes grew heavy as Jonathan chauffeured me back. We transferred me back to the bed, where I drifted off to sleep almost immediately.

Less than a half hour later, a young woman woke me up. She introduced herself as Debbie and informed me that it was time for our occupational therapy session. Still groggy from the first round, I was transferred yet again to my chair and she took me back down to the gym where we found space on a blue mat. Debbie gave me the same pitch almost verbatim as Jonathan had given earlier. "As I manipulate your arm passively, simply think and visualize the hand and arms making the motions from your brain. Our goal here is to reconnect the signal from your brain down through your shoulder, arms, and fingers. Even if the fingers and wrist do not move, just try to concentrate on how the muscles should be responding. It's going to be frustrating, but in time the signals from the brain should begin to reconnect down through the arms and into your wrist and fingers." She noticed immediately that my right side was anything but precise in its movements. However, the signal from brain to limb was certainly intact. She had positive words of affirmation that together we were going to get my upper body refiring one way or another. It was a bit redundant of the pre-battle speech from two hours earlier, but I appreciated those fighting words of inspiration immensely. Debbie's approach seemed similar to Jonathan's, focusing on weight bearing and specific muscle stretches. Once again, the fatigue set in rapidly as the hour-long session drew to a close. Both arms were beyond the point of utter exhaustion when we were finished. My left wrist locked completely as a result of the strain. There was no gauge at this point to feed off of, but something told me that she was amazed/concerned at the tone in my wrist, upper arm, and pectoral muscle. My entire left side began to spasm and shake profusely in protest to her control. She knew that we overdid it on our first day. She could tell that a slight frustration had come over me as we once again transferred me to my chair and set off back to my room.

Again, my brain switched over to a tired yet inquisitive demeanor. "What is all this shaking about?" I asked. "When they brought me here last week, my body shook uncontrollably when the cold air overwhelmed me. My arm and leg shake uncontrollably at times. This can't be normal, correct?" She then began to transfer me back into my bed. She got me situated. "You seem to have very high amounts of tone and spasticity, which is causing the tightness and then the spasms. The brain doesn't understand what to do when force is applied to the muscles. Therefore, the natural response is to clench with all its might. This is why your wrist is locked as it is for now. We will work to reduce the tone so the brain doesn't have to fight as hard to make typical movements, as it did before the injury. The proper terminology for the tone that you're experiencing is called clonus. This may subside within a couple weeks or we may look into other methods to decrease the tone—it may impact your therapy. We'll keep our eye on it for a couple weeks." "Fair enough," I said.

Author's Note:

I especially liked Debbie's approach to her profession. She was really good at her job and I picked up on her passion immediately. There are two characteristics about Deb that always stood out to me. A) She always spoke to me at eye level when explaining and teaching. Her demeanor made me feel as if she was talking to her friend, not her patient. She knew almost immediately that we were going to work well together. She also appreciated my dedication to the recovery progress. B) She took time to get to know me (I mean genuinely know me), including how she showed empathy toward Christy in understanding this colossal twist in life in a newly wedded state. The two of us would work at my journey for several months to follow, but from very early on, she didn't need a file of generic patient evaluation sheets to figure out what my goals were or who I was as a person. Each and every day that Debbie and I worked together in the OT unit, we made progress, which started from the inside believing in the process and working its way out toward physical improvements. On days when I felt really strong, she would spend the extra time with me on an array of different exercises and activities. And the days when I was frustrated or down, we'd talk through my feelings while she pulled back on an aggressive physical session. She became my advocate as well as a friend, which I desperately needed.

* * *

Lunch was served shortly after returning from the gym, and I was so exhausted from the morning's sessions that my appetite was non-existent. Looking at my whiteboard before my eyes sank shut again, there was still one more session planned for the day. I groaned in protest. I thought, "If they drag my paralyzed ass back down to gym again, I'm going to fall asleep right on one of those mats that where they tortured me throughout the morning." The nurse came in to fetch my tray and get me ready for the speech pathologist who would be arriving any minute now. She was not thrilled in the least that I had not touched my lunch due to an acute feeling of sleep deprivation, yet I believe she secretly understood my nonverbal cues as she left my dessert and beverage behind as an afternoon snack.

Another professional approached my door with an array of technical equipment transported on a mobile table. She introduced herself as Tara, and she would be working with me as my speech therapist. We exchanged pleasantries along with an overview of what my first day so far had entailed. She immediately boosted my spirits by telling me that a majority of our sessions would be conducted right here in the comfort of my room. Tara's approach to evaluating my areas of improvement was more technological than PT and OT. Hearing, speaking, breathing, chewing, and cognitive functionality were all tested. To this point, I didn't feel that these senses had been affected by the stroke. And, for the most, they were not. However, she did notice that my mouth muscles had been impacted by my noticeable facial droop, and likely some memory functionality had been affected as well. She explained that, during our sessions, we would set a baseline, and then build out a series of exercises and activities to target affected areas. As with Debbie, I could tell immediately that Tara was gifted at her occupation. Her bedside manner was impeccably empathetic and caring. She had a genuine personality with a touch of self-deprecating humor, which goes a long way when working with a patient going through a life-changing medical condition. She worked my personal goals into her daily agenda. The exercises were spontaneous and never redundant in nature. We'd get off track in conversation from time to time (usually with me relating some insane tale of shenanigans from my past). "If you're talking, we're doing therapy," was her approach to speech pathology. She was cool, hip, and treated me as a person and not a patient.

By the time that Christy arrived after work, I was just waking from my third bout of sleep. Both my bones and brain felt lethargic and weak. Even though Dr. Urs did not drop by my room, the nurses did come in to update her on my first day of therapy, which I personally chalked up as a success. My wife and I further caught up with each other, and shortly thereafter she assisted the evening staff in getting me showered and ready for a well-deserved night's sleep. We lay in my bed and watched television briefly before I dozed off.

* * *

And this is how a routine began to evolve over the course of the next few weeks. Every morning, I was woken, medicated, dressed, breakfast was served, and therapy would begin for the day. During the day, the therapists would wheel me to the gym. On certain days, specialist visits were ordered and conducted by neurological doctors, caseworkers, orthopedic specialists, as well as other specialty staff. Every evening, Christy would arrive at my room after work no matter how tired or overwhelmed she was to visit for at least a couple of hours. Sometimes she would bring dinner for us to share together. She then would help the staff prepare me for bed, and after her departure the staff would deliver my concoction of medication—consisting of painkillers, seizure management pills, and blood thinners.

A routine limb assessment conducted by yours truly began each morning as I attempted to concentrate rigorously to lift, stretch, and wiggle each extremity by power of brain function. The right arm remained weak, yet started to show noticeable progress. My fingers rebounded from a numbing state of weakness to being able to slowly move. The thought of being able to hold a pen steady enough to write or having the strength to lift an empty food service tray was out of the question. Still, the noticeable progress became encouraging and uplifting. The left side would be sure to wake up soon, I kept telling myself. Seeing as how I was practically bedridden, judging the response of the right leg was different. Though the muscles were far too weak to walk or even stand, I would test the limb with small leg raises and toe examination exercises. The left side, however, showed no sign of physical movement as I would wince my eyes tight, trying to get the circuits between brain and limb to function properly. The frustration in not understanding the intricacies by which the brain commands the specific limb to carry out its function was beyond words. Almost every professional entering the room would be hit with the same question of, "When will my arms and legs work again?" And the answer remained short and broad, making sure not to give a false sense of hope. Yet this was why they'd brought me here—to reconnect those signals while getting better.

After those first weeks of evaluating and testing, the findings in each therapist's and doctor's report aligned: They all went something like this: "We don't come upon patients of Jonathan's age and attitude very much in this facility. His therapists find it to be 'a breath of fresh air' to work with him. He has stated his vision clearly in that he wants very much to get back to his everyday living routine as soon as possible. Furthermore, he is committed and willing to get the most out of his rehabilitation here. He wants to get back home to his wife. He wants to get back to his office and his coworkers as well. He remains very committed to getting his hands mobile enough to play his guitar and his legs strong enough to snowboard come the first snowfall of next year. He has grandiose visions of pursuing entrepreneurial ventures in the future. He is very much a goal-driven individual and will thrive here with that sort of vision and attitude."

Well, what can I say? I wanted them all to understand my mindset in being here. This whole huge mess was completely fucked! Yes, I get it, folks! Every one of the evaluations that I'd been given over the past ten days had some sort of encrypted twisted questioning, asking shit such as: "Have you recently felt depressed or lonely? Do you feel that you have friends or loved ones that you can talk to? Do you have trouble sleeping because of stress? Do you worry about your financial stability while being in the hospital? Do you feel that you have let your family down? Do you feel safe in your current environment?" And all sorts of other goofy shit.

Listen, I knew within two days of therapy at the gym at the end of the hall that my type is not common here. Yet, I needed to make the best out of an insane set of circumstances. Point being was that I was seriously banged up and they all knew it! But as my dad used to say, "Make chicken salad out of chicken shit!" And that was what I set out to do here. It was my job to make myself better. And honestly, I really enjoyed the company around me. My therapists were great and understanding. I felt in good hands with the doctors here. The nursing staff treated me as one of their own. If they were going to throw me into a rehabilitation ward, this was the one!

One exciting bit of news that we received from the doctors the next week was that the incision had healed well enough that my staples were ready to come out. That freaking headdress was start-ing to show its tattered signs of battle, and, to make matters worse, the wrap was becoming terribly itchy. So, the next morning, Doctor Urs and his assistant asked for my morning therapy sessions to be held back. When they arrived with a toolbox—which consisted of a pair of forceps and likely a standard screwdriver (to act as a fulcrum of sorts)—to remove the steel sutures out of my head, I had no clue as to what to expect. I remember Christy being there, likely part out of personal curiosity and part out of moral support. You see, what they all failed to tell me before putting me under was that they were about to shave a significant portion of my hair on the right side where the skull was to be removed. Now, I'm not sure if this was an insignifi-cant detail that was skated over in the debriefing the night before or if a little bird sent the message to the powers that be to make no mention to yours truly of this pre-scalping exercise that was to be carried out. Regardless, it never crossed my mind that they needed to shave part of my head. People who know me best may tell you that I'm a bit of a diva when it comes to my personal look and fashion (and trust me, it has grown far worse over the years). But to remove my hair as if they were carrying out my execution by means of the electric chair would have seemed an absurd act of rudeness. So, as the doctors began unwrapping the bandage, I was quite keyed up to see the inner ruins that lay beneath the battered gauze. First to say, it was unbelievable how much gauze they had applied post-surgery. They must have used ten yards of the wrapping. As the sheets of cloth were removed with delicacy, you could feel the anticipation in the room begin to grow. The final layers were removed, and then the wound was exposed.

I felt the sensation of chilled air draft over the exposed area imme-diately. A silence fell over the room. Dr. Urs spoke first. "The surgeon did a very impressive job in stapling and suppressing the wound," he announced and his assistant concurred. After a couple minutes of probing and nodding, they were both in agreement that indeed the staples were ready to come out. And so they began. The procedure hurt far less than I had anticipated, which was a relief. After the medical team checked everything out properly, I demanded a mirror to see the results. Within a few minutes, my request was honored and a nurse returned to my room with a large handheld mirror. Christy sat on the bed to my left side and raised the mirror so I could see my reflection. I turned my head to the left and lined up the angle. The gash was huge! My stomach sank into a pit of nerves and disbelief. Everyone in the room paused to witness my reaction. The incision began two inches above my right eyebrow and stretched to my hairline behind my right ear. A large portion of the right hemisphere was shaved to the scalp. The sight was grotesque. There were no words. The room felt heavy as my eyes drew away from the mirror and dropped to my paralyzed arm. They all knew what I felt.

At some point in my fifth week, I asked Christy to bring two specific items from home to my room—hair clippers and my current journal that left off at Robert Wood Johnson the night before my surgery.

In a grand attempt to boost my morale, I asked Dr. Urs if I had permission to rock a Mohawk, seeing as one side of my head was practically finished already. "So long as you mind the sensitive, still-healing scar on the side of your cranium, have at it!" He chuckled and rolled his eyes as he left the room. Christy and the nurses set up a makeshift beauty parlor. Within a half hour, the masterpiece was complete (sort of my mantra to Sid Vicious, Robert DeNiro in *Taxi Driver*, and perhaps a subtle fuck-you to Berman, who had prescribed screwing with my hair as well as blasting out half of my body).

The request for the journal was straightforward. Even though my sight was still a bit blurry and the right hand was still slowly gaining back basic motor skills, I could reminisce at my earlier writings and at least make note of my current surroundings. Debbie and I were trying some writing exercises in my occupational sessions. She knew that it was important for me to have the ability to jot my thoughts down on paper. My right arm and fingers still remained extremely weak. My handwriting was horrendous and borderline illegible due to the weak grip from the fingers. A kindergarten student could likely lap me in a penmanship competition, but there was nothing I could do but work on my right-hand strength as much as possible. My right arm was the only extremity that showed signs of improvement to this point.

First and Second journal entries post-surgery

The words are hardly legible and I was likely in a heavily medicated state. I'll try my best to transcribe.

Journal Entry: March 10, 2006

"I'm still a little foggy": So from Robert Wood Johnson to JFK medical in Edison they brought me for physical therapy. I feel pretty good. I'm getting a lot of movement back in my left side (denial, clueless, and definitely medicated!). Katie and Mom are here. I get tired quickly. I have track marks all over my arms from IVs. I look less like a patient and more like Nikki Sixx. I'm working hard as hell to get back to work. It's going to be a long road.

Journal Entry: March 16, 2006

Tomorrow will be Sunday the sixteenth and that will make three weeks that I have been in medical confinement. Improvement is slow and steady and I still feel better every day. I watched the Johnny Cash movie with Spike [Makenzie] and Christy today and all it wanted to tell me is to pick up the machine and play. You wait till you see the songs I come up with after this shit. I just want to be with my wife, play my guitars, and work forever. Gotta recover though. So until I strum a note, keep working hard. I've got a shit load to work on.

///

By this point, the amount of public outreach in terms of people learning of my story was incredible. Every day that I'd return to my room from therapy, there would be cards, care packages, and notes of wellness from all over. Now, granted, I get it. I know a lot of people. But this outpouring of concern and love was incredible. The feeling was overwhelming—similar to when Dad died five years earlier. Everyone wanted to help out in some way but didn't know how. Friends, family, schools, churches, past employers, past girlfriends, past band mates all caught wind of the situation. Keep in mind that this was before social media exploded, so most of the updates on my condition were passed through phone, text, and word of mouth. Each night, Christy would open cards and unpack boxes of get-well treasures that would brighten my mood no matter whose names were attached to the gesture. My room slowly transformed into a studio apartment as boxes and envelopes showed up each day. As appreciative as I was of the kind thoughts and prayers, I struggled knowing that people were so worried about my state of well-being. Yes, this was a very serious situation that I found myself in, but it would all work itself out somehow.

Everyone from my offices (both local as well as corporate) was incredibly supportive in the weeks that followed—especially my reps Greg, Bobby, Kevin, Amber, and Mike. They knew how badly I wanted to get back to work. They could sense the frustration that only so much could get accomplished via a hospital bed. Also, I was forewarned regularly not to focus on my work but rather on my recovery. It wasn't as though I was being stubborn in regard to my therapy goals or anything, but not enough time had passed for the weight of the situation to sink in. The mentality still remained that I was going to be all better in a month or so and I'd be walking out of here good as new. I chose to block out all reality.

As always, I was especially excited when Doug, Leon, or both came to see me. They would sometimes sit in on my therapy sessions. And though grueling at times, it made me proud that they knew how hard I was working to get back to the office in short order. One morning, they both came in just to chat about day-to-day business. After a few minutes of catch-up, Doug took hold of the conversation. "Jonathan, we understand how hard you're working to get better in here. And that's awesome to see because obviously you've been through so much and you're a fighter. But we need to move on as a company while you need to get better in the time that you have here." They both watched as my heart sank to my stomach. "We plan to promote Greg to your role effective immediately until we have a better understanding as to how long it will take you to make as much of a recovery as possible. You need to focus on yourself while you're here, not the business. Not right now, at least." His words ripped through me like a dagger in the chest. There were no words. There was simply self-pity and misunderstanding. But I knew how they had played the move as well. They certainly discussed the scenario with Christy and possibly even my doctors. The feelings of betrayal and abandonment began to rise deep within. My heart filled with hurt while my swollen head filled with confusion. "Guys, I'm going to get better! I promise, I will be back in no time!" But it was already decided. It seemed to be a unanimous opinion that I was concentrating far too much on my job and not on the therapy that I was admitted here to receive. Doug then added, "Do you understand what we're telling you?" I forced myself to look into his eyes and replied, "Yes." The feeling hurt something awful. We finished up and they were on their way. In no way did I think that they were breaking ties with me, but this pain was something far different than the physical hurt I had gotten used to. I was in a state of disbelief. That day, I was not my high-energy, typical self. All the therapists and staff noticed my emotional state. Usually, I was so tired from my sessions that sleep came easily. That night was different. I tossed and turned into the early morning as all sorts of different conclusions and scenarios played out in my head.

For three straight weeks, my day-to-day routine pressed on in a mental versus physical game of chess, as I never really knew what the following day would bring from a therapy standpoint. What I was starting to come to terms with was that the excitement in achieving a full recovery I'd felt when I first arrived began to wane. My PT and OT sessions, which had started with a focus on strengthening and reconnecting the signals between brain and limbs, slowly shifted toward adapting to a life where full functionality might return very slowly or perhaps not at all. Now, granted, they never told me that directly, but I took mental note of the direction of my sessions. Cognitively, I was making great strides and we all could tell that the stroke had not impacted that particular area of the brain. However, the physical damage had been done and the prognosis of state, speed, or length of recovery was unknown. Each professional's personal outlook of my condition differed substantially from one to the other. And even though I appreciated the positive and motivational bullshit spin, I preferred the honest read of what this all was going to look like once I got out of here. And this specific thought is what slowly began to saturate long hours of my day: "What is my life going to be like if they can't get me better? I can't possibly live a normal life this way." The thought frightened me something awful. All the different scenarios played out in my head. "If I ever learn to walk again, what if I fall? What if I have another stroke? What if I black out from a seizure?" These were all scenarios that ripped through my mind.

My mentality shifted yet again as a sense of survival began to slowly take hold. As long as I remained in the hospital, I would remain safe. When the time came to leave, though, the world was going to feel dreadfully different. A major fail on my part was that I never conveyed the way I felt to staff or even family. The thought was far too much to process, but still, I couldn't shake the weight of this reality. During my therapy sessions, I would ask the therapists to experiment with different sets of scenarios and challenges. Again, they appreciated my focus toward making a full recovery while having the foresight to realize that certain aspects of my day-to-day routine would shift dramatically at some point.

It was also around this time that my therapist began experimenting with teaching me to walk again. The first challenge to overcome was yet another hurdle that the stroke had inflicted—this one in the form of foot-drop. My left foot muscles no longer had the ability to move on their own, causing dropfoot. And when these muscles are impacted, the foot has no way to function or balance in a normal manner. I was fitted with a foot brace called an AFO (Ankle Foot Orthesis), which flattened my foot while providing support to the ankle. My original AFO supplied by the hospital was approximately two sizes too big for my size nine feet. Christy had to buy me size eleven sneakers so that the plastic around my impacted foot would fit into the shoe. Simply stated, the results were simple. On my functional right leg, I had to wear sneakers that were two full sizes too big. On the left, well, we had no idea if the brace would work or not, especially until I was properly fitted by an orthotist. Down at the gym, they would position my wheelchair in between the parallel bars. With the help of one to two additional PTs, they would get me upright and work on leg exercises to begin building strength. The feeling on my right side was surprisingly normal, and with support, I actually could bear a fair amount of weight.

The left was a far different animal. It reminded me of being on ice skates for the first time at a young age. The leg felt like Jell-O, having no control whatsoever on an unfamiliar surface. Furthermore, the rapid fatigue sent my entire left side into a state of spasticity that felt like an earthquake pouring through my body uncontrollably. The initial weight-bearing leg sessions were over in a matter of minutes due to strain and intense fatigue. My right leg would overcompensate for the left almost immediately when pressure was applied to the affected side. Further complicating matters, the leg would snap and lock into place at the kneecap, making any sort of gait control practically impossible. The first few actual steps between the parallel bars looked like Frankenstein, complete with the enormous chilling incision. Though those small steps were anything but graceful, they represented large steps of progress from when I had first arrived. I intend not to steal any thunder from Neil Armstrong, but you get the picture.

If you're a survivor, you'll likely hear this benchmark phrase approximately fifty times within the first month of recovery: "Every stroke is different." And furthermore: "Every survivor views and adapts to their individual situation differently." Several studies throughout the years have been carried out on impacted arm and leg recovery. Doctors, scientists, and psychologists agree that when it comes to paralysis, the leg is likely to recover the fastest, followed by speech, followed by hand/arm. And why is this? Because use of one's legs gives a sense of independence. You need these limbs functional to stand, walk, and get from point A to point B unaided. The second is speech. Without vocal communication, what happens? You must rely on others who know you best to express thought and emotion effectively. Third is occupational or hand gestures and movements. Do you need your arms and hands for certain tasks? Of course! But methods of compensation come in many forms.

The reason I bring this all up is that, by this point, I had been bed- and wheelchair ridden for over a month. My slight speech and cognitive weaknesses were making steady progress while my arm was too far off from making any noticeable gains. When they finally got me upright and passively moving, the light bulb came on. To get my legs back to a semi-functional state would give me the independence that I so desperately craved. Furthermore, attempting to walk showed a tangible sign that I was indeed getting better. My body was actually healing and responding. Physical therapy became a huge deal to me. My main goal was to work on leg strengthening. In one week, I went from taking minute steps between parallel bars to upgrading to a large four-pronged cane. Granted, there was a pile of trial and error, slips, trips, and falls as I was forced to relearn leg-to-eye coordination from scratch. The simple task of taking a single step with the left leg had to be stripped down, then rebuilt, focusing on every fine detail that one would never actively ponder while going about everyday life. It would take me two to three minutes to stumble five yards, trying to force my brain to compute each intricate detail of putting the affected leg directly in front of the other and then repeating the task over and over again. At times my brain would reach a point of fatigue faster than the leg. I refused to let this frustrate me. When the leg or mind grew tired, I'd let myself rest, just as the therapists instructed. Very slowly, the repetition of my gait started to take form, like learning to shape guitar chords together in a fluid manner to create a melody, which morphs into the construction of a song. The nurses would let me practice my cadence under light supervision in the long hallways during the evenings so long as I held on to the railings. I didn't have the courage or the stamina to venture very far, and so my wheelchair was always close by. But these jaunts served two important purposes: One, they gave me that small piece of independence that I so desired and, two, they showed the entire staff how committed I was to getting better in here. They began to feed off of my energy, pointing out my efforts to other patients who lacked drive and determination to get better. And, yes, I had some really tough days and nights, especially trying to figure out what the future held for me. I would break down in tears at times by myself at the frustration and uncertainty of it all, which hung over me like a thick, dark cloud. I remained pretty honest with the staff and Christy when it came to my mental state, but let's face it, they had no idea what the struggle really felt like. How could they? The part of the equation that I likely didn't convey properly was that I was simply scared shitless as to what I was going to do if I ever got out of there. What I will say now is that talking those feelings out (to the proper set of ears) would have been helpful.

At some point, a state of institutionalization started to set in. My therapists and doctors were pleased with my positive attitude and progress, and the entire staff of the floor pretty much waited on me hand and foot. I had built a sense of community in spite of my condition within these walls. I was appointed somewhat of a mayor status from the nursing station. I would glide the halls in my wheelchair or practice walking from my room to the gym at the end of the hall while periodically dropping into other rooms to say hello and act neighborly. I also recall a couple times when nurses would ask me if I would pay a visit to certain patients if they seemed down or hadn't had visitors for a spell. I'd immediately put my volunteer cap on and spring (OK, perhaps "spring" may be rather aggressive), but I certainly enjoyed opportunities to engage with fellow patients. I mean, let's face the facts—we were all stuck in there together.

Eventually, there came an important meeting with my assigned caseworker. There were several topics of discussion, but two key bullet points stood out. First and foremost was my state of recovery. Yes, the therapists knew that I was working hard at my recovery, but the goal of a rehabilitation hospital is to rehabilitate a patient to regain a satisfactory quality of life. As I saw it, my quality of life had been stripped from me from the moment that they drilled my skull open and unsuccessfully screwed it back together again. Point being that I was in no way even remotely close to being ready to have a discussion about an exit strategy, and Christy and I knew it.

The next caveat was insurance. We learned quickly that insurance companies (no matter how good the coverage is) want the patient released the moment that the doctors see significant signs of improvement, especially in a rehabilitation hospital. Well, define "significant" in a case such as mine! Is it significant if I can hobble down a hallway assisted by humans with the use of a cane? Is it "significant" if I need an aide to transfer me out of bed, dress me, bathe me, and assist me with use of the toilet? Or is it deemed "significant" that I can barely pick up a fork with my "good arm" to feed myself? Neither here nor there, my caseworker assured us that she would plead with the insurance company to keep me here as long as possible. That being said, though, she was warning us that my time here was going to run out at some point. This reality sent shivers down my spine. Another noticeable shift in treatment was that my therapists were starting to conduct the majority of my sessions downstairs in the outpatient therapy gym. This was a much larger space with different machines and workout devices. I kind of got the feeling that the other therapists were eyeing me just a bit down there thinking, "If I could get my hands on him, I'd make improvements in his condition," potentially trying to one-up the therapists from the upstairs inpatient floors. Nonetheless, the reality was that, at some point in the foreseeable future, they would send me home. My caseworker further instructed me not to be concerned (or get my hopes up, for that matter) about being discharged. "You and your family will have plenty of time to make proper arrangements prior to discharge," she explained. My initial concern had nothing to do with "proper arrangements" whatsoever; the real question was—what were the next steps after I got out of there? The sheer thought frightened me big-time. The reality was, I never spoke of my concern with what was going to happen once they shipped me out of there. I didn't want staff or my family to know that this concern overwhelmed me. On the one hand, it would be a great feeling to get me settled in at home. On the other, the thought kept me awake at night. "I can't even get up or down a flight of stairs," I thought. "How the hell am I going to function in day-to-day life? Am I going to be bedridden or couchbound for my remaining days on this planet?" Hell, I had no clue as to what the future looked like.

Personally, I enjoyed the change of scenery in the outpatient gym. They had long hallways with handrails down there where I could practice walking thirty yards or so at a clip, which actually helped me form a rhythm in the reconstruction of my gait. There seemed to be everyday people in the gym as well who would come and go as their therapy sessions came and went. The environment was far more upbeat than the acute-care vibe upstairs.

Since I had built some strong relationships with my assigned team of therapists by this point, I started to interrogate them individually for a few moments at a time before, after, or even during sessions to piece together what the exit strategy looked like once the demands of the insurance company conglomerates kicked in. It didn't take all that long for them to provide me with the blueprints to the jail so that when it was my time to bust out, I'd at least have my ducks in a row. And what was leaked was actually positive news. What I gathered was that, once I was discharged, I would begin out-patient rehab here at the hospital as well as their satellite locations if I qualified for additional services. This was a great relief knowing that I could continue my PT, OT, and speech therapy sessions here. Hell, I was now getting to know the staff down there anyway so in theory it would be a great transition whenever they decided to give me the boot from upstairs.

And sure enough, that's exactly what went down on week eight upon our next meeting with my caseworker. She explained the for-mula as best she could of how the insurance companies give you so many days of inpatient care versus outpatient care. The plan of action was that she could fight for another two weeks of inpatient coverage at the max. From there we would make the proper arrange-ments to send me home and coordinate with the outpatient depart-ment to pick up my therapy right where we'd left off. The meeting details were immediately handed over to Dr. Urs and the powers that be who were in charge of my care on the third floor. From there, my therapy shifted tone to a one-on-one classroom setting on "how to survive on your own." The "what to and what not to do" in all sorts of different situations and settings. And, of course, some of these drills were basic common sense, but now, as each day passed, a strong sense of urgency set in, not only for me, but for Christy as well. All sorts of arrangements needed to be made at the house before my arrival. The two big tasks on the PT side consisted of standing up from a lying down position (in case of a fall) and maneuvering up and down steps in a safe manner, neither of which was an easy task when dealing with left-side paralysis.

Let's just say that piles of trial and error were endured in those final days. Due to the immense spasticity in the left leg as well as the brain's immediate impulse for the kneecap to lock in fear, making my way up and down stairs was borderline impossible. To make matters worse, I began "vaulting" on my left side when taking a step, which is quite common in my situation. Therefore, my gait was atrocious as I began to walk slightly longer distances with the assistance of my four-pronged cane. I walked those halls looking something like Frankenstein or the Tin Man from *The Wizard of Oz* (take your pick).

As for my arm, very slight signs of improvement were visible. If I tried with all of my might, the limp would move maybe two inches at most, like shifting a two-by-four connected at the shoulder back and forth. My weak yet partially functional right arm would compensate for the left in an uncontrollable fashion. Then the spasticity would set in due to fatigue, which would make the arm bounce up and down for minutes at a time. Multiple finger and wrist stretching exercises were performed in an attempt to prevent the tendons from shortening due to atrophy, but the spasticity was simply too much to break. My damaged brain only understood the impulse to clench down with all its might. The therapists in other departments and specialties got involved in those final days of inpatient life after convectional devices such as splints and braces proved to be ineffective to break the tone. At some point, someone came up with the idea to cast my arm with my wrist being flexed upwards for a few days just to attempt to break the spasticity. Four other professionals not including the orthopedist worked to carry out the casting. The pain was brutal in trying to position the wrist while assuring that the fingers remained straightened to maximize the stretch. My brain fought the contortion exercise like an aggravated tiger shark out of water until fatigue finally took hold enough to move the body parts into the desired position for casting. Once the job was complete, professionals wanted to see if I could handle the pain in my tendons over a forty-eight-hour stint. Of course, I immediately asked for an array of Sharpie markers and began decorating the casting with anarchy symbols and indie and punk band graffiti. Coupled with my crafted Mohawk, it caused people to wonder if I was a patient, an inmate at the East Jersey State Prison, or an attendee at a Lollapalooza concert. The sleeve was extremely uncomfortable, hot, itchy, and most of all, a bear to sleep with due to its configuration. However, I made it through the duration and the molding was cut off two days later. My OT, Debbie, tried to put a positive spin on the experiment, but the reality was that it did little to suppress the spasms, so it was back to the drawing board.

The next day, my discharge date was announced by Dr. Urs and his team. They were sending me home in two days. What I gathered was that everyone on my rehabilitation staff had to sign off on my release, stating that they felt I was "rehabilitated to the best of their ability," which they had no problem saying; they all knew that I would be reporting to outpatient therapy downstairs in the days after discharge. This procedure was obviously put in place for liability reasons. So there was a mad dash to get me through this process. On Christy's end, mounds of paperwork needed to be signed off on, not to mention instructional sessions given by the staff on how to properly transfer me, operate the medical devices, administer my medication, and know what to do if any catastrophe arose at home. It was all organized chaos to the tenth degree right up to the bitter end.

And then, the evening came. They started boxing up my belongings as I sifted through hordes of cards and care packages and gifts from so many kindhearted folks who had taken the time to send their thoughts and prayers and love over the past two months. As I recall, it was quite an overwhelming exercise in reflection. As I made my rounds in the halls that evening, I took notice of rooms of patients who had been in there for a while versus the ones who had not. The reality of an ICU unit of a rehabilitation hospital is that you can tell that there are far more long-term patients there than ones who pass through for only a few days. Hell, a few of the rooms had more personal swag than some Manhattan apartments I've visited. I visited one final time with a few of my fellow inpatient friends along with a pit stop at the nurses' station to give hugs and goodbyes and thank-yous to the evening staff. I slowly strolled back to my room to find bare walls and shelves that earlier had been littered with cards and pictures of my friends.

As the time came to settle in to bed for one final night's rest, a profusion of thoughts and emotions ran through me. The main thought on my mind was how nice it would feel to sleep in my own bed again. The second was how refreshing it would be to use our own shower. And third, how in the hell was I going to get back to the typical routine that I had before all this nonsense occurred? This was going to be bad! Christy was just trying to get back to her everyday workflow, and now she'd have to balance that while jockeying around my therapy schedule and worrying about me alone at the house while she wasn't there? This was never going to fly, I thought. There was no manual for all of this drastic change. The resources are slim to none as far as what to expect once a survivor returns home. One therapist in those final days at the hospital made the statement to us, "Well, think of it as bringing a newborn baby home for the first time." I knew that was a complete bullshit statement. The number of scenarios that could go wrong in the current environment far outweighed the positives. All sorts of negative situations played out in my head. In here I was protected from most anything. Starting tomorrow, that was all going to change.

The next morning came and one last breakfast and check of vitals was given along with my morning concoction of medication. The official time of discharge was set for one o'clock, when Christy would pick me up. A few small administrative details were still to be taken care of too. The biggest shock of the morning came when a nurse rolled in a big square contraption with a chair mounted to the top. She told me to sit up out of bed to be transferred over to the chair. I complied. "What is this thing?" I asked. "It's a scale," she stated. "We need to weigh you for our final reports." "Sure," I said. And after she calibrated the device to the correct setting, she hit the button. My jaw nearly hit the floor! In big red lights, the screen halted at 195 pounds. "Well, there is no way in hell that's right!" I announced in an aggressive demeanor as she slid me off the chair and back onto my bed. The result of this final collection of data was seriously mind blowing! And then I started to think back to when I was first admitted to Robert Wood Johnson. In here, we were told we had to eat upon arrival to keep our energy levels up. In Robert Wood Johnson, eating was something to do. When you're in a hospital, it's easy to eat a solid three meals no matter if you're a picky eater or not. It's all comfort food in this environment. The whole ritual kills time while giving you something to look forward to. The fact that Christy is a great cook and my friends would constantly bring in delicious external contraband obviously did not help my cause. I'd always had a rather scrawny yet athletic type of frame. Never had I weighed a pound more than 175, and for a five-foot ten-inch male, that was normal. This was absurdity! In my former body, a week's worth of running three or four miles or hitting the slopes for a few days would shed the unwanted pounds right off. (I've always been a bit of a weight-conscious priss like that.) But what was I to do now? I could barely get out of bed by myself, for crying out loud. Yet, for now, a petty weight breakdown was going to have to take a back seat to more important events.

Christy arrived shortly after noon and the final details of my discharge were tended to. A nurse oversaw her assisting me with the transfer from the bed to the wheelchair one final time with professional supervision. As I was carted out of my room and past the nurses' station, I thanked everyone and assured them that I would drop by to visit and show them my progress in the weeks to come. It was when the elevator opened on the main level that I felt the rush hit. As one would expect, part of me was ecstatic to get home and away from this environment of the sick and Ill fated. But an overwhelming sense of fear took hold as we moved down the long corridor and past the admissions offices, which were just ahead of those automatic doors.

I had spent a total of fifty-eight days under the care of these professionals. And now the world spoke to me in an entirely different way. Everyone who was involved in my recovery efforts did the very best they could to get me to where I was at this particular moment from a physical standpoint. How I faced the adversity that I was up against was up to me now.

Yet as we rolled out the doors, passing others going in, I couldn't help but wonder why they were coming here. I suppose they were wondering the same about me leaving via a wheelchair being pushed by a woman. "I wonder what happened to him; he looks so young," one might think in passing. Christy moved me to the side of the portico in a safe spot where she could go fetch the vehicle. In those moments, I watched an ambulance pull up and offload a person in a bed exactly as they had with me when I arrived here. I immediately was inquisitive as to what their story or circumstance was for coming here. That is simply how my mind reacts anytime I see a patient or ambulance.

13

MOONSHINER

t was when Christy swung her SUV around to pick me up that the first setbacks began set in. In physical therapy, they trained me how to transfer into a far lower sitting vehicle than her Hyundai Santa Fe. The difference in inches of swinging my left hip, then leg, up and in was critical. The transfer was an extremely challenging balancing act, which likely should have been monitored by a staff member who discharged me. Then, moments later, she was faced with the task of breaking down my wheelchair properly in that drop-off and loading area presented its own set of challenges as I hopelessly watched her struggle from the front passenger seat. As we pulled away from the hospital, the tense feeling in my gut set in and the overall feeling was extremely bittersweet.

On the way home, I had a fierce hankering for "non-hospital fare," so we dropped by the local Taco Bell drive-through to pick up lunch.

My job from the navigator chair was to put the bags of food between my legs for stability until we got home. When we pulled into the parking lot and into our designated space, Christy had to reassemble the wheelchair, then transfer me from the passenger seat to the chair (which was a far easier task than the fiasco at the hospital had been). We got me loaded up and she put the bags of food on my lap (again, my responsibility was to hold down the bags until we got upstairs to our unit). What we realized immediately was that pushing a chair with 195 pounds of dead weight is one thing within the halls of a hospital, but pushing the payload on an asphalt surface is much more difficult. We got to the curb leading up to the entry point door, then realized that the handicapped ramp had a slight gap in the transition. She tried a few times to clear the transition up to the sidewalk chair facing forward, but the smaller front wheels couldn't make it.. Finally, she moved me back to gain momentum. Upon contact, the chair cleared the gap but my arms and hands could not secure the bags of food. The whole fucking bag smashed onto the cement. The result was nacho trays and soft tacos hitting the ground and causing one hell of a mess. Christy was beyond frustrated. I was useless in the moment. I felt extremely bad and didn't say much about the incident. She wedged me through the door and onto the elevator, which barely fit us both in the cab due to the width of my chair. It was a very uncomfortable twenty-second ride up to the second floor, both physically and emotionally.

One "minor" detail that I forgot to mention earlier is that we put our house on the market a few weeks before all of this mayhem went down—right before I left for our office Vegas extravaganza, to be specific. After we got married, Christy had the full intention of getting a dog, and to make this happen, we needed a house with a yard. This all took place at the height of the Tri State housing bubble so we unloaded the Milltown pad to buy a single-family home, making a nice profit on the unit. While all my medical insanity was going on, our realtor did a great job in keeping the deal from falling apart.

In the couple weeks prior to my leaving the hospital, Christy (when she wasn't with me) would spend her evenings packing up our things in anticipation of the move. She had debriefed me on her progress from my hospital bedside, but the reality hit when she opened the door to our home, which I hadn't seen in over two months. The smell of home comforted me immensely, but the stacks upon stacks of boxes in the entryway and living room were a bit overwhelming. Christy had done a great job of clearing space between the entryway, living room, and staircase up to the bedrooms among what seemed like hundreds of boxes. We ate what Taco Bell goodies survived the impact. All in all, I was very fatigued from the pilgrimage, yet it felt so good to get home. The next order of business a few hours later was to get me up those steps to our bedroom for shower and bed. I gazed at that staircase in a way that I had never looked at a flight of stairs before. Unease poured over me as I analyzed the steepness and pitch.

In therapy, my practice of stairs (both ascending and descending) was carefully monitored and controlled by multiple therapists. I made sure that I was thorough in detail when I explained the layout of our current home, forecasting potential problems with only one able body to provide assistance. The problem was that the staff was also aware that we were moving into our new home a couple weeks after I was discharged. So the focus shifted away from the old home to the configuration of the new. Well, this was a crucial misread on everyone's part as I was soon going to learn. The only positive was that the staircase had a railing on the right side. "This doesn't have to be graceful by any means. Just get up there without falling." I did my best to relax my nerves. Sure enough, on the first step, the uncontrollable leg shaking kicked in. My left leg sensed the fear and began spasming uncontrollably. Christy drew closer from behind, putting her hand on my back for both support and comfort. With each step taken upwards, the shaking grew more intense with an engrained fear of falling back. There was no stability to be had and my balance was nonexistent on the left. I clung to the railing so tightly that grip marks were likely engraved.

The top five steps were the worst. I had never held a fear of heights, but now my body felt the threat of falling. The sensation of panic was indescribable. If I happened to fall sideways or backwards from this height, the consequences would be terrible. The summit was finally reached; my brain and limbs had completely exhausted themselves. Christy got me over to our bed as quickly as possible and I collapsed in fatigue. A task that used to take fifteen seconds now took between five and ten minutes. This was absurd! I had it in my head that I wasn't returning downstairs for days after that trip.

Twenty minutes later, Christy prepped me for the shower. The shuffle into the bathroom was manageable. What wasn't was the two-inch lip that separated the bathroom floor from the walk-in shower. After multiple failed attempts, she had to manually lift my leg over the partition. I sat on the showering bench that the hospital provided me and let the soothing water hit my face. In my enjoyment of taking my own shower for the first time in ages, I looked to my right to see my wife dowsed in water and irritation as she dove for a towel to dry herself off. The amazing feeling of taking my first shower in the comfort of my own home was instantly shattered by the guilt that I held for what I had just put my wife through. I put my head down in defeat while trying to clean myself the best I could. After she got me to bed and made me comfortable, I was drained. It felt great to lie in my own bed.

The following days were filled with adjustment, frustration, and angst. I remember not wanting to leave our bedroom mainly out of sheer dread of the staircase. I had a bed and a bathroom up there and that was pretty much all I needed during the day when Christy was at work. I had my four-pronged cane to get around if need be and there was not a chance in hell that I was going to get adventurous in attempting to scale the stairs by myself. It wasn't the best of scenarios, but at least I could keep myself content up there. Well, she wasn't having any of that. She demanded that a morning routine was carried out just like in the hospital. All I wanted to do was sleep (I mean, what was the point of getting out of bed in this condition?). She was hard on me from the start now that I was home. I was to dress myself, brush my teeth, and groom accordingly. Then we would get me down those dreaded stairs and into the living room where a couch, television, journals, phone, my wheelchair, and cane were close by. She would situate a tray next to me and fix lunch with a drink and snacks to get me through until she got home. I couldn't believe that she was going to let me stay here alone for multiple hours. Was this supposed to be some sort of tough love abandonment exercise? I had no idea. What I realized quickly was that when that front door closed behind her as she left to start her day, a blanket of fear swept over me. And the day's depression wasn't far behind.

In the hospital, there was always a pulse. There was the routine of therapy sessions and doctors checking in and meals being served and visitation hours. There was little downtime, and when you had some, you typically slept. If I got immensely bored (especially on weekends), I would roam the halls, which helped me work on my walking and balance but also served as a means of interaction with both patients and staff. And trust me when I say that I'm well known for requiring adequate doses of social stimulation on a regular basis. When you're in the hospital, there's this bizarre feeling that you're all part of this members club that's formed from floor to floor if you stick around long enough. It's a club that no one wants to be in, of course, because no one wants to be in there in the first place, but you're all sick in there together so you might as well make the best of the shit circumstances. Everybody is on the same team in there. And you only win by getting out through mere survival, an upswing in health, or rehabilitation. That's just about it.

But when you get back into your normal surroundings and come to find out that they're not nearly as normal as they once were, that's when the true sadness sets in. I remember this time very clearly, and it took me a long while to realize that it's all right to have these feelings in the aftermath of a traumatic event. All of the different scenarios play out in your head at first. But the main disbelief that racked my bruised mind now became—how was it possible that I had walked out the front door in perfect health and at the peak of my game that morning two months earlier only to now return through that same door feeling like a diseased cripple? I naturally blamed Berman and myself for most of it. Anyway, those first couple of weeks were tough for both Christy and me. The house was in shambles as we awaited the closing on the new house, and I was completely inept and a burden to my wife as she continued to pack up while I sat there in my wheelchair, utterly useless.

We had a tough time getting me settled in, as I recall. Everything was up in the air. The timing of my homecoming, the approaching house closing, getting all of my medical appointments (and there were several of them) lined up, and her work schedule—this couldn't have come at a worse time. It's one of those perfect storm scenarios when the timing would never be flawless, but we had to push forward in our lives. I felt her patience draining rapidly with me. Perhaps it was best that we were starting over in a different home. Maybe somehow this would put the events of the past few months behind us. I typically find a way to put a positive spin on less than stellar situations. This was one of those times.

Over the next couple of weeks, I reached out to some of my Bellmeade and local Philly crew to ask for a few able bodies to assist with the move. Of course, I called three, and eight showed up. Some of these guys I hadn't seen since before I was admitted into the hospital after the car wreck. It was great seeing the boys and I think that they enjoyed helping a brother out in a time of need.

14

NATURAL BEAUTY

The new house turned out to be a blessing in disguise. Though I had to deal with yet another staircase to reach the bedrooms, the layout was spacious and far better for my situation. We got settled in nicely just in time for my first round of outpatient therapy. The doctor's order was to attend therapy at JFK four days a week for the entire summer. We tried to spread out my sessions so that Christy would drop me off before work and then pick me up at the end of her day. Yes, those were excruciatingly long days, with lengthy spells of downtime in the outpatient gym, but we made the most out of the arrangements put in place. The state of New Jersey approved me for short-term disability, which held off some of the financial stress of the household. I adapted to my new surroundings as best I could. All of my therapists knew my story and how dedicated I was to my recovery. The recovery process remained very slow. I cried a lot in those first few months. I don't know if a true state of depression ever set in, but I can tell you by reading back through my journals that the frustration in my head and heart was very real. At my request, all of my guitars, amplifiers, and equipment were stowed away so I didn't have to reflect on the disability that had taken my favorite hobby away. So was my collection of 250 or so compact discs that were arranged in specific shelving beside the television, stereo, and DVD player (this was all before iPods, iPads, mp3 players, Apple music, and iPhones became the craze). It was so mentally draining to think of listening to the music that had encapsulated me before this event of catastrophic proportion tore at my life. I remember throwing a recently purchased Uncle Tupelo album (*No Depression*, which is sort of ironic looking back) into the player that I had picked up in the weeks leading up to the car accident. I had been tinkering around with one of the tracks ("Whiskey Bottle") on my own because the intro pulled me in almost instantly. The acoustic version sounded absolutely incredible and I fell in love with the arrangement. I didn't listen much past that intro when the profound recent memory of me laying down the chord structure months earlier catapulted my emotional state into an overwhelming sobbing meltdown. Christy bolted from the kitchen to see what was the matter. She turned off the player and I cried in her arms harder than I ever knew how, remembering how much I bonded with my guitars that now were unplayable. The feelings that surfaced were of self-pity and angst. No therapist, doctor, or even wife could appreciate the magnitude of having the things that bring joy to your life stripped from you by no fault of your own. Common folk don't understand the mental anguish that occurs—not unless you've been there. Although I had an incredible network of individuals who were there for me, in this war, I was alone.

Journal Entry: April 30, 2006

Approximately day 75 post-surgery: When your life becomes a cage that restricts your body, you appreciate the smaller things so much more. Gripping a guitar, tying a shoe, washing my hands. At the moment, I have very limited capability to perform these tasks. I think the word "rehabilitation" is put in place to give people like me false hope. It's a complex word that has a medical tick to it. I am not rehabilitated. I will never be free from this disease. I'll probably die from this in the long run. My brain is paralyzed and I don't know anyone who has gone through this. God doesn't have mercy. Mercy is a word for pastors and holy people. I'm fine without mercy. I've worked for what I have. I don't need a free handout of mercy. Either I'm worthy of it or not. That's not my decision. God, I'm tired. Look at my face. It is exhausted from the sick and love and hard work to get better. There has got to be a better path to my life. I'm going to die. I'm too fucking young to die.

//

And Christy didn't give up on the blasted dog idea either. The rational approach of "Do you understand what is going on around us at the moment?" and "Is this really the time to throw a dog into the mix of our chaos right now?" carried not an ounce of weight when brought up at our dinner table discussions. Hell, I might as well have gone into the patch of woods behind the house and stated my concern to a random hemlock or pine. There was no use in delivering my opinion on the subject. Her mind was made up. She found a legit breeding establishment back in Pennsylvania, and before I knew it, she loaded me into her vehicle, cane and all. And I knew better than to voice my opinion on the way out, so I inserted Wilco's *Yankee Hotel Foxtrot* into the CD player and napped for the duration. But she knew what was on my mind. If memory serves, not much conversation was drummed up on the way there as I peacefully protested what was about to go down.

However, if you have ever seen a golden retriever puppy at a mere eight weeks old, it will make your heart melt. I tried to fight a good fight but lost in the end. He was absolutely precious as

he slept in my lap the entire way back to Jersey. I forced myself
not to make eye contact with Christy just so she couldn't gloat in
my reaction. For some reason, she put me in charge of choosing
a name for the little shit as long as it was something within the
parameters of reason. It didn't take long for me to choose his sur-
name also. I named him Marshall James after my idolized guitar
prodigy Jimi Hendrix (proper, in reverse order), which I thought
was fitting for the cause. And, of course, he fit in like a glove to our
little family dynamic. No rules applied to the little prince either.
Any form of no sleeping in our bed or no sitting on the furniture
was evaporated within roughly six hours of bringing him home. He
loved sleeping above our heads as well, which I never understood
but reluctantly tolerated. Within a couple of weeks, I realized the
role that he played around the house. He was a companion to me
during the day when Christy was at work and he gave me a sense
of responsibility in a time where I felt that all responsibility had
been stripped from me. Marshall gave me a sense of well-being
during a period when my self-worth had been stolen. He relied on
me. Christy saw the relationship between a dog and his sick dad
flourish with genuine love and joint dependency, which we both
needed. He served as my medical response dog even if his purpose
was simply to lift my psychological well-being. She made the correct decision to bring him into our lives when she did.

Since the beginning of this whole mess, Doug and Leon had kept
close tabs on what was going on. The whole office would visit me
often and the heavy cloud of not being with my work colleagues
hung heavy as those dog days of summer passed by. I fretted and
journaled sporadically about what the future held for me professionally. My goals remained steady, but there was no real game plan in
place. The team of outpatient professionals who now managed my
care wouldn't even entertain the idea of me returning to work anytime remotely soon. Sometimes, I'd ask Doug to come with me to
therapy so he and my doctor could track and discuss my progress in
recovery.

Journal Entry: May 18, 2006

Approximately 100 days post-surgery. It's something early like 8:30 A.M. I dreamed about work last night. I miss all of it. I miss the rush of the game. So the question becomes, when will this run its course? All I want to do is put a guitar in my hand but I can't. Listening to music is further crippling at the moment. I want the creation piece. I've been in this stage for close to four months. When you're sick and laid up like this, it feels like an eternity. I don't deserve this. No one deserves this. Someone wake my arm up! Someone give me a sporting chance! This is bad shit. I don't belong here. I have paid my dues. Don't destroy my life. I'll make something big out of this. I promise you.

And let's just say that I wasn't exactly on board with the outpatient rehabilitation department's approach to my case either. (But more on that in a moment.) A panel of professionals took the approach of, "Because of Jonathan's age, we intend to "throw the kitchen sink at him" in a grandiose attempt to either motivate me or set me straight on their vision of how to rehabilitate a type A personality such as mine. I truly hadn't a clue as to their intention. Everybody was on board with my outgoing, positive attitude toward my therapy goals. Yet this state of mind didn't fit in with their typical patient wellness agenda. I was the exception to the rule, and I was wise enough to realize quickly that they were throwing spaghetti at the wall with my case.

Two specific incidents shifted my view.

They explained to Christy and myself that they wanted me to meet with an in-house psychologist twice a week. I balked at this suggestion immediately. "Does this "therapist" have a TBI as well?" I spat off. "No, of course not," was the response. "Well, then how in the hell is a psychiatrist going to understand what I'm going through?" This was my brilliant logic. Furthermore, they concocted the idea to send me to a cognitive therapy program at an off-site facility of theirs. They claimed that in order to release me back into the workforce I needed to complete this bogus program. I knew immediately that this was complete and utter bullshit! Christy was irritated with my pushback to the staff. I was not buying into this plan of action and held my ground.

As for the PT, OT, and speech sessions, my progress was moving along to plan. All of my therapists and I were on the same page when it came to the short- and long-term outlook. On the physical side, my left leg was starting to build stability and strength. I began to push away from my wheelchair and out into the world as my walking and ability to climb and descend ramps and stairs improved. This was a big win in terms of my therapy goals. On days that I didn't have therapy, Christy let me take short walks around the adjoining neighborhood (as long as I took my 4-pronged cane) to work on building endurance as well as gaining my footing on natural surfaces such as grass, shale, concrete, and pavement. Just to get out of the house during the day was a great boost to my psyche. In the mornings and evenings, Marshall and I would hang out in the backyard and wooded area behind the house. We both enjoyed going into the woods and exploring as my leg responded to an array of different surfaces and obstacles. He simply wrestled with branches five times his size, played in piles of leaves, and rolled in mounds of random filth for which we would catch hell for, once back inside the house.

During one of my first mornings in outpatient therapy, Dr Escaldi, who took over as my outpatient doctor, had a man-to-man conversation with me. I had good rapport with the guy right off the bat, so the conversation was well received. He began, "Listen, we all know that your situation is very different than most in here. It's my job to provide you with all of the resources that we have available for the time that you're here with us. We can't force you to participate in any one area of therapy, but my expertise as well as intuition tells me that you want to make the most of your resources here." I picked up on what he was inferring immediately. He wanted me to have an evaluation with the in-house psychologist who held office hours on-site. He also wanted me to take a second evaluation for the cognitive program as well. "Listen, Doc," I said, calm and appreciative about this candid dialogue between us. "The last thing that I want to convey here is that I'm a bad sport. You also don't need some pompous son-of-a-bitch such as myself trying to tell you how to do your job. However, my psychological well-being is certainly intact. Put yourself in my shoes. Sure, I'm going to have my down days. It all comes with the territory. And as far as my cognitive state goes, I've heard about the program over there at the other campus. None of that seems to resonate with my physical recovery, which is the main issue here."

"Will you just try what I recommend?" Escaldi solicited again. "The psychiatric piece is simply an evaluation protocol for most patients here. If the meetings don't help, you can let us know and we'll cancel them. The cognitive piece is far more intrusive than we can provide over here. Again, you can opt out, but I strongly suggest that you take the evaluation over there," Escaldi explained. "Sure." I collapsed and then agreed with his suggestion. "What can I lose?" At least the guy shot straight with me. His demeanor was eye to eye, a professional-to-patient pep talk. The conversation was appreciated on both ends.

15

RADIO-FRIENDLY
UNIT SHIFTER

L ater that week, the psychologist sessions were scheduled. I had noticed her a few times before slipping in and out of her office, which was located in the main outpatient gym. The trusted professionals who worked with me gave up a brief bio on her. They told me that she called upon patients between the multiple facilities within the hospital network. They also inferred that she was neither a socialite nor team player amongst her fellow staff. She was coined as the "professional misfit" of the outpatient team. And yes, the first time I laid eyes on her, I could see that she had the personality of a tire iron. On the morning that she came to the general waiting area in the gym to scarf me up for our first session, I looked her sharply in the eyes and extended my right arm, giving her the courtesy of a firm handshake. I then followed her into her office.

You could tell instantly that she had been debriefed about me, and I read in her eyes that she wasn't about to put up with any of my malarkey. Yet I was keeping my end of the bargain with Escaldi. Her resting bitch face told her whole story. She looked like she had been permanently damaged by a parochial school system while never living up to her clique of choice in postsecondary education. Her office was dark, fitting her character, with a large green chair positioned in the center of the dimly light room. She gestured to the plush recliner, which was my cue to be seated. I acquainted myself with the room as she closed the door and took her position in another chair some ten feet away from mine. She gave me a few moments to take in my surroundings. I noticed this small tabletop waterfall contraption, which was used to calm the mood. I'd seen it in movies. It was all so hokey that I almost burst out laughing at the absurdity of it all. But I remained astute.

She began with what I'm sure was her typical scripted rhetoric. "So, what brings you here today?"

Hold on, right off the bat lady—let's stop for a moment. What sort of fucking absurd question is this to lead in with? I can't recall if I kicked back, slacking in posture, or began cracking my knuckles profusely in agitation, as already I was about to become unglued.

She continued, "And what do you want to get out of our sessions, and how are you adapting to life at home?" I played along, keeping a humble frame of mind as she drew up a slew of questions and scenarios. The minutes on my watch dragged along as I checked the hands obsessively. Of course, she inquired about my apparent anxiety along with my intentional lack of focus. I also began to refer to myself in the third person at some point, which, I had a strong hunch, pissed her off immensely.

Then she finally did ask an emphatic question that actually did hit home and was worthwhile of discussion. She asked, "How did you feel from the time that you got here to the hospital until the day that you left?" I had written about this often throughout these months and had much to say on the subject matter. But I needed a bit more from her before I could trust her. Within moments, I became the interviewer. She felt the movement of the pendulum. I could see it in her expression. So I shifted in my chair and leaned into her to engage completely. "Do you really want to know how I felt those days in the hospital?" I began. "Have you ever stayed in a hospital for an extended period of time?" I asked. "No, I have not," she stated. "Well, have you ever watched the movie *Shawshank Redemption*, by chance?" I inquired. "No, I haven't," she replied. "If you watch that film, we can have an impactful conversation about your question because I've written about the subject in great detail," I said.

She glared back at me in discontent. "I have not and likely will not," she spouted back, trying desperately to regain traction from behind the wheel. "I'm not saying you have to watch it tonight or this week, for that matter," I said. "Just when you get a chance, at your leisure, and then we can discuss in detail." I positioned my request. "It's an award-winning film in which certain themes from within overlay precisely to how I feel about the question you just asked," I added, about ready to blow a gasket at her demeanor. "I don't have the time for that sort of activity," she replied. I was finished bartering with this shrew! I shrugged my only functioning shoulder and said, "So be it, then."

We both agreed to end the session right then and there. I remained polite and courteous as I left the office, but I was boiling inside, and I got the sense that several members of the staff were anxiously anticipating what I had to say upon my exit of that office. One could feel the thousand-pound gorilla in the gymnasium the minute that door cracked open. Her intuition likely warned her that I had positioned myself just so back in the waiting area, and her instinct was correct! As the wench left that office roughly five minutes later, she hauled past me, being sure with all her might not to make eye contact. My demeaning eyes locked on her presence like a cheetah's fangs on a gazelle. "What a fucking phony rat," burned through my head at that moment. Her irritation with me was certainly reciprocated as she walked out of the room. The mood quickly lifted in the gym. My OT, Debbie, was the first to flag down my attention with her eyes. She was working with another patient at the time or one of us would have immediately gone to the other for an impromptu debriefing, which was what they were all waiting for. But I was sure they already knew the outcome of this session.

Next on the list of asinine professional recommendations was attending an eight-week (three times a week) cognitive therapy program. I did my part, going through the gamut of a full-day on-site evaluation, which I got suckered into committing to against my will. I pleaded with Christy and my family that this environment would have little impact to my long-term recovery. But they weren't having it. The entire arrangement was a train wreck to begin with. Christy would have to drop me off at 7:15 A.M. to get to her work by eight via the New Jersey Turnpike, which I knew was a complete beating for her. Then she would have to fight traffic northbound back up to Edison to pick me up after five. This was not a positive scenario any which way you dressed it.

On my first day of cognitive therapy, they were anticipating my arrival. The first order of business was to meet with another senior caseworker type, whom I had met weeks earlier during the evaluation. I walked into his office to find him buried behind mounds of loose paperwork and files stacked in multiple piles upon his desk and the credenza behind him. The whole room looked like utter chaos. And this is coming from one of the most disorganized, fly-by-the-seat-of-your-pants individuals to ever walk the earth, so you get where I'm going here. I sat down in the one chair that wasn't littered with paper as he began to rummage through multiple stacks to locate (what I'm assuming) was my file. The obese as well as disorganized bloke opened the file and began to mumble incoherent remarks to himself in between his enormous gasps for oxygen as I waited patiently for the meeting to formally begin. Then he started with his opening remarks. "So, I'm not really sure as to why you're here given your high functionality level. We had to go up in the attic and dust off some old materials given that we typically don't see people like you in this sort of program." I didn't know if he was serious or trying to add lame humor to the absurdity of the statement. My mouth nearly hit the floor as my blood began to boil. "Well, then, what the holy hell am I doing here for Christ's sake?" I cursed back like an enraged hyena infected with rabies. "This is exactly what I have said all along! My cognitive functionality was the very least of my problems when you look at the situation as a whole. They told me that this program would help prepare me for getting back to work." "Well, we will do what we can and see how this goes," he told me with a pathetic shrug of confidence.

Now, to this day, I'm not actually sure where to put the blame. My doctors, my therapists, the outpatient caseworker who was assigned to me, or those corrupt insurance providers, perhaps. This was complete and utter sabotage to my recovery as I saw it. I was not even supposed to be here. A whole slew of obstacles began to take shape as I began my sessions. First off, they promised us that I still would be attending physical therapy at this facility. What a flipping joke that was. The physical therapist that I was assigned may have been better suited as a cafeteria worker or janitor. In the two sessions that I had with her, she learned far more from me than I did from her. She outright admitted it! The gym was small, dimly light, and primitive. No patient would be inspired to get better in this environment. It was completely dreary and dismal. The therapists made the experience that much worse. None of the staff that I encountered were passionate about their job. The patients also picked up on my observation, as we would discuss during lunch.

What was not mentioned to us prior to my arrival was that this particular facility was home to many severely affected traumatic brain injury patients who were now past the acute stage of recovery. Some patients lived on-site and some were brought in from all parts of the Tri State region. Within a few days at the facility, I figured out exactly what was going on in here. These patients were the most serious outcomes from very serious injuries. Several patients were my age or younger. Many of them naturally gravitated to me. I met a guy who worked in construction. A year earlier, he'd fallen off of a third-story roof and landed on his neck. I met another guy who tried to commit suicide in a hospital parking lot. His tool of intent was a twelve-gauge shotgun. When he pulled the trigger, he missed his desired target (being his head), shot the right side of his face off, and lived to tell the tale. I met a very sweet twenty-two-year-old girl who obviously came from a family of privilege. A year ago, she had gotten bucked off of her show horse, leaving her with a lower spinal cord injury. She now had very little motor control of her head, arms, and legs. My buddy Preston suffered a massive TBI from a football injury during the fall of his senior year. My other friend Chris was thrown off of his Harley-Davidson motorcycle and slammed into a stop sign. After the paramedics arrived, the county coroner was summoned due to the victim's failing vitals. Turns out, a faint heartbeat was detected and he was placed in an induced coma for six months until he eventually woke up and remembered everything except that he couldn't speak due to the nature of his brain injury. There were several other tragic cases, but those are the handful that I remember off the top of my head.

Are you getting the point here? I've never spent any time behind bars, yet I do understand the difference between general population versus solitary confinement due to mitigating circumstances. The professionals who were to keep my best interest in mind threw me to the wolves as some sort of trial and error experiment. And this was the result of lackluster professionals in my universe saying, "We're going to throw the kitchen sink at him." So what did I do you may ask? I revolted like a fucking pirate! That whole staff knew of my disposition within a couple of days when I verbally blasted a particular therapist the moment that we wrapped up her evaluation of my "memory deficits". She was at the very least bright enough to realize from the start that this was not the correct environment for a survivor of my functionality level. She knew within two sessions that her methods and skill set had no bearing on where my physical deficiencies lay. She knew that I did not need to be cognitively re-circuited. Yet I was forced to play the injured lamb while making a couple of professionals' lives downright challenging. And trust me when I say that these same superiors let me know on behalf of the entire staff that they were not pleased by my acts of piracy either. For hours at a time, I would sit by myself in the courtyard eating my lunch or journaling my thoughts between my sessions. The rest of the time, I found myself interacting with, as well as consoling, patients of all types in the common areas. Again, multiple individuals affected by injury somehow gauged that my set reason for being here was the exception to the rule. I listened to their stories and circumstances that had landed them here. I offered back as much positivity and wisdom as I could, along with a realistic perspective through the eyes of a survivor (me).

And, of course, some staff members didn't particularly like the fact that the patients were engaging me and vice versa. My thought process was that if I was going to be caged here against my will, there had to be some positive expertise that I could volunteer while the rest of this circus pulled its act together. At some point, whether week four, five, or seven, they all knew that I was just going through the motions in utter protest. And it wasn't a sense of me carrying a bad attitude on my shoulders or anything. They all knew that they had taken the wrong approach in sending me here. We were just trying to get me through the program without disturbing the patients who truly needed these sorts of resources. I never said that the program was altogether a failure; rather, this particular form of therapy was in no way a correct solution for my situation. As a matter of fact, it was borderline reckless and irresponsible for the people "who knew best" to admit me here in the first place. To set the record straight, they didn't "pull any strings to help me out," nor did they "cut through mounds of red tape" to get me enrolled into this "elite" program, and neither did they "put in a good word because this was a bit of a 'one-off' situation." If I didn't have a strong positive attitude, it could have really fucked me up to be surrounded by that degree of profound trauma. This had nothing to do with returning me to real-world scenarios nor proving that I had a certain degree of mental stability. The professionals royally screwed up on this one.

So, these were two scenarios in my recovery where the system failed us. Of course, nobody truly accepted responsibility for the mishandling of these therapy hurdles. I am a huge believer in professionals taking a holistic approach for every patient going through any sort of rehabilitation no matter what the case may be. No single method is a "fix all" solution for all patients. Even at this critical point in my journey, I knew my body and cognitive functionality well enough to know that the professional advice I was given was skewed. It all was new to me back then. We really didn't understand that I needed to become my own advocate (hell, I didn't even know what the word "advocate" meant). I had no experience with any of these avenues of therapy and modern medicine. Therefore, we took the advice that was placed before us.

I was trying to form a parallel with the psychologist when bringing up the reference of *Shawshank*. And if by chance you have not seen the film, it is an incredible depiction of the human spirit. My intent was to explain to her how prisons and hospitals have more similarities than one might think. No sane person wants to be in either facility because in some form each institution takes away one's independence. And if you're in one long enough, you begin to transform to the environment that surrounds you. As the character Red brilliantly states after hearing about the suicide of his friend once being released to the outside: "Believe what you want, the walls [prison] are funny. First you hate 'em, then you get used to 'em. Enough time passes, you get so you depend on 'em. That's 'institutionalized.'" And that is how I felt when they released me back into the world. That psychologist didn't want to head down that rabbit hole with me for whatever reason. She didn't even give me the courtesy to finish my thought. And pondering why she felt the way she did toward me is no longer important. Thinking of her now is a waste of my time.

The takeaway here to all professionals is that it means so much when you go the extra step to understand the likes, and dislikes, and fears, and goals, and triggers, of the patients that you work with. Find the person behind the patient! The demeanor and attitude of professionals means so much. So many professionals take the voluntary role of being the caregiver if only for just a short amount of time. The generosity is so appreciated in the moment, even though those that need you most don't quite realize it yet!

16

LIFE IN VAIN

My insurance permitted two more weeks of outpatient therapy following the cognitive therapy debacle. After that point, we would have exhausted all the rehabilitation for the year. All sessions following would be considered out of pocket expense. The positive was twofold. First, I was making strides in achieving my physical goals. My left leg was gaining strength. My balance was still a work in progress, but with the assistance of my cane, my body was finding new ways to compensate. My daily walking jaunts would take me close to a mile in distance. The hyper-controlled leg movements slowly started to mold into a semi-sustainable gait pattern. The left leg and the brain were consciously working together to make the signal reconnect. The efforts were in no way pretty to the typical eye, but my therapists were noticing the improvement. I was forcing my brain to recompute the leg functionality as best it knew how. They all saw the results of the extra work. I remained completely committed to my therapy goals. Small tweaks and improvements slowly mutated to larger natural advancements in my recovery.

The second win that emerged from those last few sessions was that we all agreed I could begin the process of reinstating my driver's license, which was granted after meeting with an optic specialist at Penn College of Medicine. I was back on the road. I wasn't about to give in on my "get back to work as soon as possible" mentality once I was cleared either. And, seriously, what did they expect me to do? At this point, nearly seven months post-surgery, all conventional avenues of therapy had been exhausted. My end of the bargain was fulfilled. I promised my doctors, therapists, family, friends, colleagues, and myself that I would work my ass off to gain back as much functionality as possible. This was the hand of cards that I had been dealt. Sure, over time, I was bound to see one-off improvements in certain areas, but we all knew that this was the end of the road as far as the initial cycle of conventional methods to therapy was concerned.

As I reflect on this period of time, my sense of urgency combined with intuition and street smarts kicked in. There was no way in hell that I was going to let something as illogical as a stroke set me back from adapting to a normal state of everyday life. There was also no chance that I was planning to lie on a couch all day while watching *Judge Judy* reruns and eating lunchmeat sandwiches five days a week collecting long-term disability. It simply wasn't going to happen. Doug and Leon agreed to at least entertain the idea of having me rejoin the team in some capacity. And I was grateful for this, knowing that my best bet to return to a typical workweek would be under their terms and guidance. Yet, in the back of my head, I knew that these past months had shifted the dynamic of our sales goals as well as the future significantly. I was no longer in the day-to-day operations of the organization. The landscape of the logistics business is known to change very rapidly, and I had fallen far behind in my absence. So, as a backup plan, I made a call or two to our corporate office where those folks had been rallying for my recovery from the start of this debacle—if for no other reason than I knew I could find sound professional advice from within to make the correct decision going forward. And those calls were how the seeds were planted internally of my ultimate intentions. The goal was to devise a strategy to get back into the "now" at a system level and then formulate the means to purchase either a new franchise territory from the corporate office or buy an already existing market from a franchisee looking to make an exit in the foreseeable future. To my amazement, the powers internally made a few calls on my behalf, and some chatter started floating around that I may be interested in pursuing other opportunities from within the system. As I saw things, the guys had told me months earlier that they had to move on without me while I was recuperating from surgery. Well, that made me essentially a free agent. I was flattered by the response of multiple large ownership groups who were interested in the possibility of acquiring this renowned yet beat-up soldier. The talks inspired me greatly. The business confidence that had washed away over a seven-month sabbatical was reignited. I became excited once more to regain my stature from within our organization.

Yet through all the excitement and options presented in those couple of weeks, the reality had started to set in. I was still in rough shape physically. The months of therapy had definitely delivered signs of progress, but I was in no shape to relocate or undergo some sort of massive transition. Hell, I still couldn't even drive a vehicle because I had to be officially cleared by my neurologist first. It didn't make sense, nor was a change of this magnitude fair to Christy. She had enough on her plate as it was.

At the beginning of August, it made practical sense to return to my New Jersey central office. The guys and I devised a role and strategy so that my daily workload would be far less strenuous than overseeing my full sales team. My responsibilities would shift to spending more time in the office drafting reports and monitoring customer attrition. The entire team was excited as well as relieved when news of my return was announced. I finally began to feel a sense of professional purpose again. On days when I felt up to it, I would go on customer visits with Amber just to get back out in front of our customer base. I would interject where I felt my feedback was needed, but honestly, I felt like the entire room was judging me. I became extremely self-conscious of how I carried myself in front of other people out in the professional world. The way that my left arm and shoulder drooped made me extremely uncomfortable. The ankle foot orthotic that stabilized my leg was bulky and actually prevented my gait from flowing naturally. At least with my right hand function, I could always give a solid handshake, which boosted my confidence.

My constant battle with fatigue caused more setbacks. When Kevin dropped me off from the office in the evening, I would crash onto the couch, cuddle up with Marshall, and sleep for the better part of the evening. I would sometimes skip dinner altogether. By the time we got me up the stairs, showered, and into bed, we were both wiped out. In the mornings, it felt as if Christy was getting us both ready since it was very difficult to effectively tuck my shirt in, finagle my left shoe around my brace with the use of one arm, and virtually impossible to knot a necktie correctly. A year before, we were thriving as a newlywed couple. Now it felt as though a rhythm was lost. I felt horrible as our once dynamic, lively relationship became shadowed by her caregiver responsibilities. It didn't seem fair. Yet there was nothing I could do.

Doug and Leon watched me struggle with the physical adjustments as well. I became extremely sensitive when they would walk behind me as if to gauge my progress (or lack thereof). Maneuvering up flights of stairs was still extremely taxing. My left leg would feel the tension from my brain and kick out in a roundabout swinging motion as I fought to remain relaxed while approaching any sort of incline. My movements still remained noticeably catawampus. The struggle to keep up on the day-to-day, as well as my physical abnormalities, made me even more self-conscious in the office environment. They would all go completely out of their way to help me, which was very much appreciated, yet it also made me feel coddled. They could see my frustration in my step and in my eyes. As the weeks dragged on, I started to sense the pressure internally. To this day, I'm not sure if the feeling was one of hypersensitivity on my end or if the guys were beginning to talk through some sort of permanent exit strategy for me. The signs all seemed to be there that my time had truly expired within the organization. And, just as in the hospital, the feeling of being let go was not an option in my eyes.

In multiple conversations, I explained to Christy that I had a hunch that the guys may have had second thoughts on bringing me back to the office full-time so quickly. It's that feeling that you get when you know that a particular environment suddenly feels oddly different. It's that sixth sense you get in a failing relationship when you know that the other party has checked out. I could feel it all mounting in those final couple of weeks. So I pulled my resources and internal contacts together to figure out the next move, which took roughly three phone calls and one meeting to lock down.

On the morning that I gave my intent of resignation to Doug and Leon, I had no prepared agenda. They came into my office, we sat down, and I told them what was on my mind. Looking back, I probably could have handled that conversation differently. After all, these guys were like big brothers to me. It wasn't as if I were about to slap an Americans with Disabilities lawsuit on their desks or anything. They had both guided me down an amazing career path in an organization that I was passionate about. The set of extenuating circumstances that had brought us to this point were not of our choosing. It was all shit luck, shit timing, and shit consequences. We had a few heated moments in that discussion, but in the end, we all hugged out our frustrations and I left that day without feeling excessive blame toward either side. The three of us were too far in the thick of my injury in that moment. This wasn't about changing my role or moving me into a different area of the operation. Everyone who has ever worked for those two (back then and in all of their future endeavors) will always appreciate their sense of entrepreneurial vision, importance of culture, and preposterous generosity. The adventure that they had invited me to be a part of was epic. Whenever we see one another, it's all the exact same shenanigans as if we never lost a beat. The three of us are still very close. Any shred of deception or misunderstanding from either side has been put to rest many years ago. They will always be two of my greatest mentors, both personally and professionally. Yet there was something else out there for me. Whatever the hell that looked like, I had not a clue.

Journal Entry: February 21, 2007 (1 year post-surgery)

Well, this is the reason that I did this. This is the reason why in twelfth grade I started to take my thoughts and convert them to written words in blank books. I remember writing when I got into my fraternity and when I turned twenty-one and when my dad died, and when September eleventh happened, and when Tom Stanley and I drank a bottle of chardonnay at his dining room table while he was showing me points of interest off of his map of Italy where he and Matt traveled to years back while Mrs. Stanley made us a brilliant concoction of Chicken and Stove Top casserole when I first arrived in Philadelphia. I have written about our new golden retriever Marshall and the love that my wife gave me. And how my best friends from Bellmeade came out here to see me the day before I went into surgery. I've written about sex and drugs and music. I write about the melodies that make a difference no matter who the critics are. I write of my mom and Katie and Makenzie and Jimmie Johnson and Randy McKee (Puddin' degenerate) and Preston from JFK and all my acquaintances from the JFK facility. And all this has brought me to a year ago tonight. I remember a bit about what I wrote about that night. I (we) had no idea as to what the long-term effects were going to be. I was struck with something unimaginable. And I don't know if I am beating the aftermath or simply going through the routine at this point. I am not strong nor an inspiration. I simply survived. And what I don't know at this point is if eventually I will heal or not. I will never get back to one hundred percent. I can work at it to recoup all that I can. And I don't know what to do so I've done what feels right. I kept going from the point where it stopped one year ago. I feel that I've earned this in some strange fashion. I don't regret it and I don't feel that I could do it again. I do wish that they had let me have my guitars on the last night. We simply had no idea. I will always feel that a part of me has died but I'll always fight it. I'll be who I am. I feel that I have lived the lives of three people at this young age of twenty-nine. Last year, I went to bed this night with not the slightest clue as to what my delicate future held. It is sad and now they expect me to find the positive. I'm tired and I have been for months. It would be a lot for anyone, I suppose.

Well, that last phrase from a few moments ago may be a little glib, but here was the situation. I needed to find employment immediately (to save my sanity) even though now I realized that the odds of success were weighed heavily against me. No longer could I manage at the aggressive pace that had made me effective in environments past. My body didn't have the endurance necessary to be an intensely competitive outside sales manager in a fast-paced organization. Admitting to myself that these were simple facts was the equivalent of administering the "put to sleep" injection into a three-year-old mare that was just about to hit her prime. But these were indeed the facts now and they could not be ignored. I needed to work at my own pace. I was staring down the barrel at the precise moment of the entrepreneurial leap that I had envisioned all those years. Much sound advice and guidance went into the formula and business plan. And I wasn't about to allow a single professional or doctor or therapist to advise me otherwise. This was the moment that the pivotal chess move was to be played.

In the weeks prior, I'd worked out the specifics with the corporate office to purchase the selling rights to the central Pennsylvania market, on which I had already concocted the first right of refusal. A business loan was needed to make the deal go through, so I shook down funds through a local lending establishment. The contract was signed off on November 2, which was twenty-four days before my thirtieth birthday. I had achieved my goal set back when I graduated from Penn State eight years prior.

Not everyone was excited about my new endeavor. Christy was a wreck initially when I broke the news while rocketing down Interstate 280 South toward Brunswick. She became panic-stricken almost immediately as I said in an authoritative tone that the deal was done and we were heading back home. Granted, we had been toying with the idea for months, if not years. It simply made sense to be close to family. I could feel and hear the concern in her words through the phone. What we had built out here on our own might be swiftly coming to an end. We truly loved it here in central New Jersey.

The first words out of her mouth that evening were not those of pride in a spouse or confidence in my move to action. "I am not comfortable with all of this," was her reaction as I entered our home that evening. My intuition had told me in the months leading up to the purchase that I was taking action for the betterment of our family. She was immediately nervous about selling the house, finding work comparable to her current solid career path, and the state of my health, as this sort of life-changing stress could trigger adverse effects to my recovery. These were all fair and legit concerns, and the emotions we both felt can best be described as bittersweet. She wanted to be a supportive spouse and I wanted to make the transition as seamless as possible for us. We did feel a true sense of excitement, looking back on it all. We'd accomplished what we had set out to achieve. The timing just felt right to start a new chapter. And, naturally, our family and friends were ecstatic that we were coming back to our home turf.

We frequently traveled back and forth between central Pennsylvania and New Jersey looking into our next home purchase as well as spreading the good news. It was a time of great excitement combined with exorbitant amounts of stress. The first issue that arose was that "the Great Tri State Housing Bubble" had collapsed just a few months prior to our listing the house. The economics of the housing market flipped virtually upside down and we were forced to sell our house at a substantial loss. We then purchased slightly over our budget back in State College, where a recession-proof economy in the arms of a thriving university community naturally forced the price of poker higher than what we had assumed. In the end, between the buying of the business and the sale of the New Jersey property and our purchase of a house in central Pennsylvania, we had accrued debt, which certainly was not part of the initial plan.

17

ARE YOU A HYPNOTIST??

The business model for a logistics reseller channel was pretty straightforward. It's not like I was provided with a book of business and a full-time staff or anything fancy. The majority of these offices started in the basements of parents' houses, run by entrepreneurially minded people like me. I would handle the sales part of the business, which was my area of expertise. As I naturally expected, given her impressive skill set in logistics, Christy found an opportunity to broaden her career almost immediately after we moved to State College. She would also handle the business book-keeping and financials until I grew the business enough to support additional resources. As with most any start-up venture, the learning curve was steep, especially when all parts of the operation were handled by two people. Getting any sort of traction, then stability, then profitability, is far easier said than done. Again, I was extremely self-conscious of my physical limitations at first when approaching my clients. I would go to extremes to hide my disability by jamming my left arm into my pants pocket in a vain attempt so that no one would take notice of my handicap. I would overcompensate on my walking, acting as if nothing were wrong with me. I was embarrassed by the indentation of my skull on the right side, an aftereffect of the surgery. I was embarrassed by the way my facial droop affected my smile as well. I looked like an upright train wreck. And, above it all, I was in debt for the first time in my life.

Failure was not an option. To go from a thriving office dynamic making very good coin to wandering through business parks alone with a noticeable limp schlepping freight services was a real eye-opener. I couldn't afford to pay myself for several months until a solid book of business was established. Our reserve fund from the glory days of Jersey dwindled rapidly with all the up-front expenses of the business and the new house. We both felt the financial belt tightening. We'd been used to a very comfortable quality of life during our years in Jersey. Now, I was eating one-dollar slices of pizza for lunch and sneaking flasks into public drinking establishments so we didn't have to pay for alcohol. That first year as a business owner was extremely demoralizing, to say the least. The mindset of "the grass is always greener on the other side" set in rather quickly. The feeling of being stranded on my own desert island is the feeling that comes to mind, looking back.

The saving grace was Christy, who landed a very nice employment opportunity a few weeks after we arrived in central Pennsylvania. The financial burden weighed on me heavily because, at that point, I was not pulling my weight. Our sex life became almost nonexistent, and my mindset was that the disabilities along with financial stress in the household made me feel unattractive and dispensable. Drinking our emotions away at the neighborhood watering hole among locals and phony acquaintances became the routine on weekends.

Granted, we were not in dire financial circumstances, yet the minute cracks in the lining of our relationship were becoming noticeable. My friends especially saw the shift long before I did. This was likely the natural denial phase setting in. Any entrepreneurial venture of this magnitude that I have ever gotten myself into requires a long-term mindset. The positive was that I had an impressive knowledge of the business model from front to back. The negative was that, at my age, I didn't understand the necessity of holding a significant bankroll to keep the day-to-day goings-on of life consistent without severely affecting an overall quality of existence. I had mentally prepared myself for the sacrifices necessary in the beginning stages of starting up a business like this. Whether the initial setbacks that we would likely endure were or were not addressed beforehand is truly debatable. The bottom line was that in those first few years the climb to achieving a level of financial success came slower than expected, which furthered the burden placed on our small family dynamic. And in my typical fashion, I overcompensated matters through an array of trips and adventures, attempting to deflect difficulties.

The reality was that Christy was not happy. I slowly witnessed her collapse, beginning in those first couple of years after we'd returned to State College. The evenings of her secluding herself in our bedroom for hours on end, combined with dried running mascara on her cheeks from bloodshot, swollen eyes, told the tale. On multiple occasions, her frustration point hit boiling levels, and in a few instances, she demeaned me for my physical limitations. Her words stung something awful. My father used to lay into me for the most mundane issues imaginable. Even from a young age, I used to let those words roll in one ear and out the other, knowing that the root of his dissatisfaction was typically stress induced. Yet, to hear my spouse consciously demean me in the same way my dad once had did not feel right. My feelings were hurt and I felt ashamed. Very seldom did I fire back at her though. Honestly, there was no point. It has never been in my nature to throw tantrums, or fight, or slam doors in fits of rage. By this point, the writing was on the wall. We all knew it, including our friends and families. One late afternoon after reconciliation was no longer an option, I sat her down at the kitchen table and simply asked: "What do you want and how do you want to handle it?"

The stats on divorce following a traumatic brain injury are mind blowing. One national case study found that between forty-eight to seventy-eight marriages impacted by traumatic brain injury result in divorce. I feel the explanation is twofold.

First off, there are very few resources out there in navigating stroke/TBI among couples after the acute stage ends. One can only imagine what that looked like fourteen years ago. When they wheeled me out of the hospital on the day of discharge, there wasn't really much to guide the well-being of the two of us. We had been married for six months! What is there to say? Christy and I navigated through my recovery the best that we knew how. The learning curve from a physical and psychological standpoint was immense. I left that hospital as a completely different human being. My body was obviously severely affected, yet the cognitive part of my brain was for the most part in check. This created a dangerous combination because my physical hurdles were now playing a losing game of catch-up while my outlook on life and goal setting never changed. I was not going to let a fucking stroke hold me back from living my life! It was simply not going to happen! And I know this was painful for her to watch—the day-in and day-out. And this becomes the struggle to find a balance of an everyday existence that seems so far into the unforeseeable future. This finish line of maximum recovery may as well have been established on the planet Neptune. We just had no idea. Nor did anyone. Yet when the other person feels the setback of serving as the caregiver, everything becomes scrambled and difficult. I'm sure my type A, sometimes-stubborn mentality didn't help matters either.

And, secondly, I feel that wedding vows might as well be exchanged in a Howard Johnson's parking lot because, frankly, they don't mean shit.

18

LOST CAUSE

So the questions that I hear from people are the following: Were you sad? Of course. Did you feel a sense of abandonment? Yes. Did you feel a sense of responsibility for what brought the relationship to this state of being? Yes. Did you feel ripped off and cheated on? Yes. Could you see yourself getting through this with a positive outcome? Yes. Were you a faithful husband? Yes. Did you love her? Yes. Did a sense of heartbreak set in? Well, to be perfectly honest, No. Defeat was accepted with a graceful bow-out as the months passed by. Yet, to my surprise, that painful pit in your gut when the cheerleader girl who dumps your punk ass in high school never really hit. I believe my head was telling my heart that this marriage was becoming dangerously toxic. Then survivor mentality began to set in. "What if she were not here? What would I do? How am I going to live by myself?" sort of questions began to pop up all around me.

First to say that, for the most part, this was a very amicable divorce. Our families (especially our mothers) were shell shocked by the news, but we kept the specifics fairly simple. She kept the house; I kept the business, no kids, and split custody of our golden retriever Marshall was agreed upon. In my eyes, it was the best we could do in a shit scenario. The smart decision was to move back in with my mother until affairs got sorted out. After all, the objective to moving back to central Pennsylvania was to be closer to family. Right? My mom had since moved out of Bellmeade Drive and lived roughly an hour away from State College in a town just south of Altoona. The commute from her house to the office was manageable, and sure enough, she was ecstatic to take me in after the initial buzz of the news died down. Granted, the thought of moving back in with my mom in my mid-thirties seemed less than appealing, but we made the best out of a grim set of circumstances. Besides the obvious advantages, such as prepared dinners and saving quite a bit of money with minimal personal expense, we made a bit of an adventure out of my time there to help me get my mind off of things. By this point, I had a small staff in place at the office, so my mom and I were able to take jaunts while marking off bucket list items like visiting Europe, Vegas, driving the PCH from San Francisco to San Diego, trips to South Florida. It was sort of like being at mid-thirties crisis camp when you actually have the means and funds to do crazy adventures. Everyone around me was extremely understanding and sensitive to the situation as I slowly as well as tactically broke the news to friends. Many made the extra effort to include me in all sorts of events and activities to take my mind off of the situation. And yet again, I was extremely grateful to my support network of friends and family who were there to lift me up at a time when I felt down because of yet another huge setback.

One other pertinent point to mention was that I made a commitment to myself to reengage in physical therapy. I found a local outpatient facility. I very much wanted to explore options out there for strength training as well as gait function for my leg. Of course, the staff at the clinic was blown away at the tale of my journey. They tried the best they could to push me with new techniques, but it amounted to the same outpatient programs that I had enrolled in after leaving JFK outpatient in New Jersey three years earlier. My functionality was not in line with the patients (mainly elderly and sports injury) that the clinic usually treated. The staff admitted that I was essentially teaching them more than they were teaching me. However, the massive plus was that I'd gained access to a gym adjacent to the physical therapy wing. I simply figured that if professional guidance was no longer an option, I could at least strength-train on my own. And that became my routine, which has carried on to this day. The stationary bike, elliptical, floor weight machines, yoga balls, three-mile daily walks, and nutritious eating habits became my day-to-day routine. I hadn't been happy with my body ever since that last day in the hospital when they had the nerve to weigh me. Now marked the time for change. I wanted a different body and a different outlook on life. And my weight indeed began to drop after a few weeks of intense exercise and adjusting my caloric intake. The scale went from approximately 190 to 145 pounds within three months. People noticed the change immediately, which was a real boost to my inner confidence. I joked to my friends that I was simply getting back to "fight weight," which got a rise out of those who supported the cause. I did get a bit carried away with the whole thing when I started looking borderline emaciated. And I learned quickly that women do not find this figure to be alluring in any capacity.

After the particulars of the divorce were ironed out, I again found myself in another goal-setting mentality. First, I needed to find a suitable house back up in State College so I could be closer to the office. The criteria for a house was simple. It needed to be affordable and all living space needed to be on the first floor. The last thing I needed at this point was to fall down a flight of stairs. It didn't take long before I found a small two-bedroom spot on the outskirts of town but still close enough to all desired amenities. The space was manageable despite my disability. It had a small yard, which I could hire a lawn service to maintain, and a paved pathway that led to a local park, which would be perfect for Marshall. I also hired a couple of Mennonite cleaning women to clean the house, do a couple loads of laundry, as well as figure out some light cooking. The entire arrangement was a great fit for my quality of life. It wasn't the perfect scenario, but the important aspects were covered. Most importantly, the house gave me the stability and peace of mind that I was moving on with my life.

The business was starting to gain momentum as well. The small one-man franchise operation consisting of myself in a pivotal sales role turned into a devoted office team. Outside sales representatives, customer service agents, office management, and freight coordinator positions were strategically onboarded to accommodate our growing customer base. It took time, and what felt like boatloads of non-expendable capital was thrown at the wall and sometimes out the window. My commitment to reinvest as much as possible to pay off the bank and build out a solid staff started to come to fruition. The machine was finally oiled properly to make a solid run in growing the market out while sustaining our current customer base. It certainly wasn't the ten-cylinder engine from New Jersey Central or multiple other powerhouse markets throughout the system, but we created a buzz nonetheless as our numbers climbed from one million to two million in annual revenue over the course of a year's time. It was a fun run for us as we hit our system growth numbers three years in a row and were recognized nationally for our efforts. We all fondly recall multiple team trips to Atlantic City, Pittsburgh, Philadelphia, Hollywood and Miami, Florida, as well as Christmas and dinner party extravaganzas that required a bit of explanation to our office manager when she would open the American Express statement and roll her eyes at our overblown behavior. My offices always held a "work hard/play hard" slogan. And the State College market was true to form. I've always felt that a solid in-house team builds a strong sense of office culture from the inside out. It was essentially a three-year curve of hiring well and firing well (with a couple exceptions along the way). There were times when I thought we would never get the equation correct due to hiring struggles in a secondary market. Yet it somehow came together.

It was right around the sixth year after the surgery when I finally took a step back to take an audit of my recovery. Feelings of penned-up hostility, frustration, and anger toward the situation as a whole began to dissipate. Where I had once owned an extremely carefree, jovial personality, self-consciousness now overpowered the way I walked, the way my arm hung, and how my fist stayed locked in a permanent position. There were times when I would be out and about running errands or dining when I'd come across my reflection in a window or in a men's restroom; my immediate reaction would be to feel dismal about the way I carried myself. Or how people would stare awkwardly on a wedding reception dance floor when I was just doing my best to fit in. And of course it's hard to get used to knowing that people are talking about your medical situation behind your back all the time. It's all of those "one-off" moments when I had feelings of shame and awkwardness. And even worse, I would stew and fret about certain environments in my downtime—how could I compensate better within my surroundings and master certain scenarios? When contemplated repeatedly, as was the case with me, these gut feelings and questions could make a person go mad. I was so critical about how others judged me, especially when I first started to go out in public again. It truly was a long struggle to feel a sense of normalcy in those first few years. But then, almost magically, I came to a sort of closure where my insecurities regarding my physical setbacks vanished. And I became myself again. A massive weight of both embarrassment and struggle was lifted from my shoulders.

My saving superpower was that I tried to remain optimistic and fight the fight to keep a consistent quality of life. I tried to be strategic about how I could manage on my own. I came up with all sorts of ways to cook, drive, cut grass, cross a street, climb up and down staircases, open a ketchup packet with my teeth, open a jar or unscrew a bottle by logging an object in between my left bicep and armpit for stability then twisting with the right hand, balance a pizza box with one arm while forcing the door open with the other, shower, shovel snow, hang clothes rather than fold them, dress properly, navigate stadium seating, and just learn to ask for help when needed. Those are some of the "day-to-day street smarts" that you pick up when living your life with a disability. It's tough for anyone else to decipher the right and wrong way of accomplishing a task so long as the task is completed in a safe manner. It's sort of the "walk a mile in my shoes" mentality, I suppose. Through local medical channels, I was invited to attend and speak at multiple stroke and traumatic brain injury groups. Medical device companies pertaining to TBI caught wind of my progress as well. Though my age set me apart in some ways, the stories I heard in these group meetings were completely in line with my struggles. And the more survivors that I interacted with, the more I realized just how similar our experiences were. We all were doing our damnedest to pull resources together to help one another. In the first few weeks post-surgery, everyone was telling me repeatedly that every stroke is different. I agreed with them with a tongue-in-cheek, blow-them-off attitude. Yet when I started interacting with other survivors on a personal level, well, it all finally sank in. And, of course, I wanted to do more.

Dealing with the aftermath of paralysis never truly goes away. Do you adapt? Yes, to a degree, eventually, but the challenges are both mental and physical, which is the toughest part of the whole mess. Every single day brings a new set of challenges from the moment you get out of bed. My surroundings have to constantly be analyzed all hours of the day. For example, before I get out of bed, I need to make sure my eyes are focused and adjusted to the light. Then, when I stand up, my feet need to be grounded correctly, ensuring proper balance while fighting through the left leg spasticity. Before I get in the shower, I need to make the bed and lay out proper clothing attire for the day. After carefully stepping into the shower (using a properly enforced shower rod to assist in the transition), I need to again ensure that my feet and body are anchored into position to prevent a fall. And, furthermore, I need to situate the bath mats correctly before entering so that the floor doesn't get wet upon exit. Any given day's activities, excursions, and adventures must be thought through at a high level before being acted on.

Going out and about in public is a completely different animal. Maneuvering through office buildings, grocery stores, restaurants, hotels, public transportation, theaters, music venues, sports complexes, airports, and inclement weather requires a unique approach of forecasting and calculation. These thought processes become extremely challenging, especially when you are gifted with a completely non-attention-to-detail mentality such as myself, both pre- and post-stroke.

The positive here is that, over time, patterns begin to develop. Routine will reform for those who commit to getting back as much of a quality of life as possible. And the best part is that if your lifestyle was not healthy or fulfilling before your injury, this is a great time to hit the reset button. Rewire your mindset!

As the seventh anniversary of my surgery approached, I started toying around with the idea of somehow documenting my journey of recovery. Of course, my personal journals were a great way to track my progress, and they also served as a form of mental therapy as I put my thoughts, goals, achievements, and frustrations to paper. But could I do more? As I began putting myself into the community of survivors, one reoccurring theme was mentioned over and over. There were not enough resources available to help all those impacted by traumatic brain injury, stroke, paralysis, and beyond.

A buddy of mine and I were half brainstorming, half bullshitting one evening over drinks when he asked me if I knew what blogging was. My response was that I hadn't a clue. He explained that it's a website that serves as an informational platform, written in an often chronological journal style. He had been dabbling on a blog of his own that showcased a comic strip character he'd created. He further explained that adding content was neither labor intensive nor overly taxing to my "nontechnological" nature. As I pondered the potential opportunities for using this type of media, a single thought bounced through my brain like a pinball—namely, that I could use my journey over the past five years to inspire others going through any sort of life-altering struggle. The writing was on the wall. In so many of these groups and meetings I attended with fellow survivors and caregivers, the lack of resources became evident almost instantly. Naturally, I became more and more vocal in these organized environments, which I began to attend regularly. The groups typically consisted of between five to twenty participants and were organized by physical therapy managers or social work supervisors who I became acquainted with over time. Hospital networks with departments dedicated to stroke and traumatic brain injury began reaching out to me to speak to these groups about my journey. These were typically hour-long round-table stroke support group settings where I would discuss topics such as goal setting, positive attitude, and perseverance as I reflected back on different points of my recovery, with time allotted for Q and A afterwards. These gatherings were fairly informal in nature, being arranged in conference rooms, hospital auditoriums, cafeterias, physical therapy gyms, and lobbies. Telling my story while giving sound advice to fellow survivors and their families came rather natural to me. I truly enjoyed giving back to the impacted community that I was now part of. The time had arrived to become an advocate for myself as well as all affected by disability, no matter the shape, size, or scope.

Outstroken.com was launched publicly on February 22, 2012 to commemorate my seventh year in recovery after surgery. The underscore "Taking the Trauma Out of Traumatic Brain Injury" was added to lighten the mood just a bit. The logic was quite simple—to build out content from my everyday life post-stroke. The intention was not to bog my audience down with piles of medical statistics and points of pity. Rather, I saw it as an educational tool to inspire others with similar challenges to understand that they are not alone. We are a community together, and together we can overcome adversity no matter how severe the impact. The goal of the blog holds true to this day. The posts serve as "looking into a typical day in my life." I aim to keep the content light and positive, yet at times the topics shift tone to serious and educational in nature. And, to my amazement, people from all over the world started visiting the site. Somehow, even though I have very little knowledge of search engine optimization and such, people found out about my content. The feedback was instant and exhilarating. The sheer fact that others wanted to read about my story was baffling to me. Over the course of the first year of the launch, more than eleven hundred viewers subscribed to the site. The response was incredible. The site was nothing flashy. I didn't put thousands of dollars into fancy bells and whistles, nor did I have the technical ability to get too creative with HTML and video production. Ninety percent of the content consisted of pictures shot from an iPhone camera and short video clips of any given situation that I would encounter throughout the course of a day. It was simple. It was relevant to anyone who had dealt with adversity in life. And, on a minute level, I was capturing an audience of survivors who needed guidance while navigating the tricky waters of living life with any sort of disability. It warmed my heart knowing that my content was helping others.

19

ALL TOMORROW'S PARTIES

'm still not sure why everyone is so fascinated with my dating life once the ink on my divorce decree dried. There's nothing very saucy about it. Now, what I will state is that, yes, there may have been an exponential learning curve involved by A) being out of the game for twelve-plus years and B) well, how do you explain to a woman that half of your body is blown out and your wife left you? No red flags or baggage here! The last thing on my mind was how to put myself back on the available market (OK, perhaps not the last thing but you get the point). I had two rules after Christy and I split: First, I was going to wait for a year before I would even entertain the thought of casually dating. Second, even if I thought about throwing my line back into the pond, I wasn't going to conduct any sort of relationship in State College. The town was simply far too small for the two of us to conduct random courting appearances. Furthermore, the pickings were rather slim in a rural college town. I dreaded the thought of my former wife catching wind of me out with another woman. Yes, I get that my methodology was a bit skewed on the topic. I tried my best not to make a situation painfully tense for either of us even though she chose not to reciprocate the gesture. For the record, I was really proud of the way I carried myself as our divorce played out. At the end of the day, it was a civil split. I suppose I could have been a real scumbag and thrown women in front of her out of spite. I could have ponied up to the bar of specific drinking establishments where the social buzz of my single presence would surely have made it back to her in some capacity. But that's just not my style.

You'll likely be astonished to hear that even with the Google machine, YouTube, and online dating sites, there isn't an abundance of resources out there when it comes to strategic dating methods with someone with extreme left-side paralysis! So, once again, this all was going to be a pile of trial and error in uncharted waters. The whole thought of dating in my condition became daunting almost immediately. The problem/reality was that my self-consciousness (not to be confused with self-confidence) was the number one obstacle in casual dating. The mindset had nothing to do with all the entertaining, casual flirting and double entendres that go with the whole game of it all. Rather, I truly could not get my brain off the idea that no woman would want to be put in a position of being seen accompanying a disabled man in any sort of social situation.

The entire concept was nothing short of a fallacy. To spin it around, think of a man prancing around with a female who bore something similar to my set of physical limitations. People would stare at them thinking that he had some sort of repugnant sexual fetish of some sort. I suppose that after the last seven years of becoming used to my new series of limitations in my old skin, things had to be looked at differently. I learned to accept that. And, yes, I understand now that my logic was perhaps completely skewed. However, when you have no true point of reference, the brain will talk your self-consciousness into just about anything. All that I could think about was being rejected by society as well as the opposite sex due to a condition that was out of my control. Sure, I possessed the same charm and sense of humor that I'd held a decade earlier, yet the old swagger and confidence were now locked inside a handicapped state of being. And this crushed me. It's partially the by-product of any divorce when you're on the losing end of the stick, I suppose. But the disability piece definitely enhanced the blow to my ego.

Eventually, they all beat me down: friends, colleagues, family, all of them. "Just throw yourself out there and see what happens," they said. "Yeah, that's easy for you all to say!" became my response. At first, I was resourceful in my approach. I told my friends that I would date by referral only (meaning, if you know of any single women out there who want to hang out, give them my story/situation and get me their digits to line up a meeting of some sort). Little did I know that pool of leads would dry up within two weeks. (What about all these friends that I talk about. Nope!)

Soon after, more strategic methods were adopted. Match, Tinder, and Plenty of Fish all fell into heavy rotation. At first, I was massively skeptical with all those dating apps and sites. So what did I do? In typical fashion, I overcorrected entirely by giving half-truths in my profiles—my justification being that I would simply explain my situation upon meeting these girls and everything would work itself out. Wrong! The backfire revealed itself almost instantly with a couple of trial-and-error meetings in the beginning of my campaign. I suppose I took the exact same approach I once had fallen into a few years back by trying my best to cover up what was ultimately out in the open. The aftermath of the stroke would always be a part of me. There was no way around the fact, and it made absolutely no sense to cover up the scars. As with any dating scenario, when you excuse yourself to use the men's room, the woman might naturally check out your build and physical features while your back is turned. I am never going to walk with a perfect gait again. My left arm will likely forever hang with my wrist remaining clenched into place. None of this is ever going to change. And so, I started desperately trying to change my image to appease the women I courted in my post-stroke infancy. The reality was that the 200 percent marked-up Prada button-down shirt, stylish pair of Seven jeans, the swanky pair of Magnanni Italian loafers, and whichever wine bar and tapas establishment that you skidded your BMW into would never change the reality that you spent two months in a hospital bed recovering from a series of unforeseen events.

In time, I began to get more comfortable with the whole racket. People didn't define me as "Jonathan, the guy with the stroke," but rather "Jonathan, the charismatic guy with a really neat story of perseverance over the past seven years while overcoming some truly mind-blowing hurdles." That had a particular ring to it that gradually built my confidence back up. To my knowledge, no woman that I pursued, dated, or courted ever broke off an engagement or felt a sense of awkwardness due to my appearance or disability. As a matter of fact, it was as if I could do cartwheels and backhand springs around some of these girls due to my 150-mile-per-hour sales guy personality loaded with the fly-by-the-seat-of-my-pants attitude toward life. On the other hand, if I was a complete screwball and they told me to hit the road, well, that was a whole different story altogether. Looking back, I have to chuckle at the two consistent inquiries that surely raced through each woman's mind before, during, or shortly after our first meeting transpired A) Did this guy sue the doctor who short circuited his brain at this age? B) Does everything work correctly down below? You know what? These questions are completely fair game when getting to know me, when personalities start to match up, when she begins to appreciate my obscure sense of humor, and when you both feel confident enough to let your guard down a little. And that's the good stuff! But yes, at times there arises that semi-awkward conversation when the atmosphere spices up and the journey to the bedroom begins. I figured out, though, that the conversation becomes only as uncomfortable as you make it out to be.

Sure, there may be a bit of trial and error involved in the beginning, but honestly, the situation finds a way to be extremely comfortable for both of us. There is nothing wrong with approaching the topic of sex up front and talking through it while not talking through it, if you catch my drift. You were likely nervous as hell when you were a curious teenager trying to figure out the opposite sex. Well, nothing really changes in the world of disability either (except perhaps the subtle shifting of a few pillows to enhance comfort).

Especially women in my life (post-stroke) have this remarkable sense of intuition when they watch me go through my everyday routine and analyze how I approach the simplest of tasks. They tend to become extremely inquisitive when analyzing my often-atypical approach to everyday scenarios. Not to say that the male gender isn't equally as intrigued by the way that I navigate various tasks as well as environments to maintain a desired quality of life without relying on others. The list runs a mile long but as they say, there are a slew of ways to skin a cat. It's the simple stuff that most don't even think about while going about the course of a typical day.

And for all those overachievers out there who want to walk a mile in my shoes, feel free to give a few of these tasks a whirl while reflecting on the challenges of overcoming paralysis adversity starting with, properly holding an infant, tucking your dress shirt in properly, putting a belt on while hitting every loop, tying your shoes, hand-signaling while riding a bicycle, sliding on your necktie with your collar down, opening a "pull" doorknob, opening a medicine bottle, opening a bottle of Listerine, opening a bottle of wine, closing a car door once sitting in the driver's seat, opening a packet of crackers, handling Saran Wrap effectively, maneuvering the toilet paper roll when the dispenser is fixed on the left side, swimming, driving a boat, operating a manual transmission, shoveling snow, jumping out of an airplane, putting a condom on, putting shams on a pillowcase, cutting food while dining, crocheting, applying deodorant effectively, tying a garbage bag, changing a light bulb, removing clothing tags, using fingernail clippers, putting on a Band-Aid, folding laundry, operating a fire extinguisher, putting a carry-on bag in the overhead bin, hanging pictures, extracting a splinter out of a finger, carrying a casserole dish, busting crab legs, peeling shrimp, opening a jar, slicing pizza, applying toothpaste to the brush, hanging a shower curtain, zipping a coat, riding an escalator, making an egg white omelet, lighting fireworks, juggling, getting through airport security, making a tight connecting flight, shooting pool, playing golf, skeet shooting, making wedding soup, breaking down a cardboard box, lighting a cigar, gardening, signing a document of any size, husking a corn stalk, skateboarding, steering a shopping cart (plug for Wegmans on this . . . Well done, folks), opening a produce bag, operating a pogo stick, effectively using an elliptical bike, running with the bulls, moving furniture, peeling an orange, making pottery on a wheel, kneading dough, manscaping, alligator wrestling, catching a football, solving a Rubik's Cube, twisting a pepper cracker, flossing, tackling a spiral staircase, lawn ticket seating at an amphitheater, taking a recycling bin to the curb, driving a boat, getting into the ocean, getting to shore once in the ocean, walking on sand, navigating on ice, getting settled in Beaver Stadium, taking a bra off, playing pinball, eating mussels, starting a tractor with a choke, getting dinner out of the oven, baiting a fishhook, applying a Biore strip to the nose (ladies, just try it!), preparing shish kabobs, dishing out ice cream, maneuvering through ATM drive-throughs, transitioning out of the back seat of a two-door vehicle, using a chain saw, double Dutch jumping rope, picking up a large takeout order, dairy farming, buffet style dining, untangling a knot out of a shoelace, putting a key on a ring, tying a bow, unwrapping a straw, opening a ketchup packet, wrapping coins, gift wrapping, striking a match, sharpening a pencil without electricity, getting biscuit dough out of that exploding twist container, using a broom and dustpan, playing an accordion, fastening a Southwest Airlines safety belt, cutting pizza with a fork, putting on a beanie, or steering a wheelbarrow.

These tasks are all attainable so long as proper thought and planning are implemented. And to conclude this segment for the curious by nature who have not properly interrogated any of the women that I have spent time with post-surgery, allow me to ease your wandering minds. First: No, I did not see the true gain in seeking financial restitution from the brain surgeon so no malpractice claims were ever filed. Second: Yes, everything functions quite strikingly within the confines of my 350% marked up designer denim!

20

MAYONNAISE

Typically, two weekends a year a crew of my Penn State fraternity brothers get together. The memories last forever. Roughly twenty years after graduating from our beloved alma mater, we have now spread out all over, yet when the stars line up on these particular weekends, the cast of characters stretch from Philadelphia, New York, Baltimore, Pittsburgh, New England, Los Angeles, Washington DC, Florida, Dallas, to points in between. Whether it's a weekend of cheering on our Nittany Lions to victory at Beaver Stadium or getting together at one of our houses in February to play poker followed by raising hell in an urban setting, the planning and anticipation leading up to these occasions is half the fun. The sheer fact that fifteen or so of us have remained such solid friends over all these years is a true testament of loyalty to our school and to one another—which is what the bond of brotherhood is all about. Keep in mind that a majority of these guys were by my side when my dad got sick, when I was in really rough shape post-surgery, and when my marriage fell apart. No matter the distance, we've remained tight.

For football weekends in Happy Valley, my bachelor pad serves as the perfect venue to host these animals with the stadium situated less than two miles away (during games you can literally hear Dean Devore announcing the action over the roar of the crowd from my driveway, which is pretty sweet). As you can imagine, we all carry on like wild hooligans during tailgates. If you have never been to a Penn State football game, you simply must put it on your bucket list! No matter the opponent, the environment is truly electrical! For the 2017 season, the boys coordinated the weekend of September 16 when our team was taking on the University of Northern Georgia (where we gave them a 56-0 spanking). We had quite the cast for this particular weekend, including our buddy Bradley who flew in from Los Angeles to participate in his first home game experience in eight years. Brad got into town on Thursday evening, and just like the last time we'd hung out in LA when I was out there on business a couple years earlier, we picked back up right where we'd left off. The evening was a blast. We caught up on our lives and pitched entre-preneurial ideas back and forth as we often do. The rest of the crew was to filter in on Friday morning as tee-off times were slated start-ing at 11:00 A.M.

The one activity that I do not participate in is the annual golf outing on Friday. The reason is quite simple. Between business obli-gations at the office, getting the house in order, and running mounds of errands, there are simply not enough hours in the day. I typically elect myself the detail of securing our gang ever so precious real estate at a downtown-watering establishment. On any given Penn State home football weekend, the town transforms blazingly from a local population of 42,000 to over 250,000 in the twenty-four hours before kickoff on Saturday afternoon. I admit that I may get a little overexcited/-consumed/-anxious with making sure schedules and timelines are followed and maintained with precise accuracy. Because once five o'clock or so hits, the turmoil begins! And throughout the course of this forty-eight-hour period, there are no wives, no girlfriends, no kids, no rules, and not a worry in the world. We are all masters of our own domain!

That is until Sunday morning hits, when the reality sets in with thumping heads and sore throats. Neither all the coffee nor orange juice on the planet will block out the fact that long drives and flights await most of these guys. With the workweek to start the following day, we always find ourselves thinking about the next time we'll do it all again.

Sunday was September 17. Apparently a couple of these fellas have wives with stringent expectations when it comes to their arrival back into Dodge. My house was basically cleared out by 9:00 A.M. What remained was the pungent smell of a house that had been ravaged for a weekend. A plethora of garbage overflowed from the trash can in the garage. And there was the litany of random beer bottles, wine bottles, half-drunk soldiers of various canned beers, makeshift ashtrays, half-eaten boxes of pizza and D.P. Dough calzones, and don't forget the beer-pong table on the back deck littered with the reminiscent display of victory and defeat. The two recycling bins dragged to the curb by two men apiece were a reflection of success or embarrassment, depending on how you wanted to look at it. Once the tornado exited central Pennsylvania, only Bradley remained. He was catching a flight back to the West Coast later that afternoon. We both sort of surveyed the situation, which two days earlier had served as a functioning dwelling. I looked at Brad, Brad looked at me, and I announced, "Fuck it! I'm going back to bed for a couple of hours. I'll clean this shithole up later. If I'm still sleeping, wake me up before you head for the airport."

Between the current condition of my house (yes, I admit that I have acquired a minor case of OCD as of late) and intending to wish Bradley off, I woke up maybe an hour and a half later and headed for the shower. I felt a wave of vertigo, so I paused for a moment to let my sense of balance catch up to my body's trajectory. That was likely the result of two too many mimosas from the previous morning, I figured, as I brushed off the episode and proceeded to the shower, which felt glorious.

By the time I got out, I could hear Brad beginning the task of putting himself together for a day of travel. I threw on the most comfortable clothes I could muster up at the moment, gearing up for a long day on the couch after my final guest's departure. I could tell that my throat was still a bit compromised from hollering at the top of my lungs in the stadium for a good duration of the football game. And then I greeted Brad once again. I don't recall what we were talking about when I noticed it, but something was definitely off with my voice.

///

Journal entry: September 17, 2017

It was PSU boys' weekend and as usual, we had a great time. We pounded Northern Georgia by four or five touchdowns. We've looked pretty damn strong in these first few pre-conference games.

I had a small scare this morning which seems to be lingering. I am not sure how to diagnose it yet. This weekend was what it always is; big party, drinking, terrible diet, slight dehydration, late nights and early mornings. All this will never change on football weekends here. Today I woke up around 8:00 and I was dizzy. Not as in hung over dizzy but more like, I was struggling with my balance. I said my goodbyes, cleared the house, and went back to bed. I woke up two hours later and noticed that from time to time I was slurring my words. Brad was still here. I could tell that I couldn't make out certain words. I took my medicine, called Amy (remember the girl from the beginning when I had aura in her swanky hotel suite? Well, there you have it!) and figured this was a symptom of pure fatigue from the last few days. Well, it's now 7:30 P.M. and not much has changed as far as I can tell. I feel fine. I just went to Lowe's to pick up a couple deck items and ate dinner. All this is in check. But it scares me a bit. I talked to Amy and struggled to put sentences together without slurring. Even my penmanship (although always anything but neat) is sluggish and dragging in my opinion. I'll see what the next couple of days bring. Without a voice, I'm toast damnit! May this just be a fluke of exhaustion and nothing more? It's nothing to screw with. No party is worth a medical setback at this point.

I remember that evening attempting to go to bed early. The problem was that I was very nervous so sleep was hard to come by. The plan was to get up early and conduct a self-exam before heading to the office. To my knowledge, there was no change. Certain words simply didn't come out correctly. It was as if my tongue would become paralyzed when conducting certain movements. The problem wasn't so much that my mind didn't know how to form a sentence, but rather that getting simple words to roll of my tongue and out of my mouth was proving to be ridiculously challenging. Regardless, I figured that this absurd flicker of meningitis or something would pass throughout the course of the day.

Journal Entry: September 18, 2017 (Morning)

I can simply tell that I am nervous by yesterday's events. I had a good night's sleep but the same vocal issues seem to be staying rooted at the moment. I took a customer service phone call this morning and I struggled at points in the conversation. It seems as though I'm becoming very nasally while trying to put together long-winded sentences. I am taking precaution to line up a neurologist. I'd rather be safe than stupid if anything goes haywire. I feel perfectly fine and intend to keep the routine going as always. I refuse to think myself into being sick! This is not how I work. I cannot tie this episode to any one event in particular. It simply was a status quo football weekend. Nothing out of the ordinary transpired so to have some sort of neurological misfire is beyond me at this point. I will proceed with caution over the next few days. This is scary. This obviously is not typical by any means. I am certainly taking this seriously and moving along with caution.

Shortly after arriving at the office, the panic started to set in. I summoned my operations manager Kyle into my office and asked him to critique my speech. He pointed out that my voice sounded a bit hoarse but noted that was likely the residual aftereffect of the weekend mania. I was nervous and immensely sidetracked. I stared out my office window at the trees and cars and people below. My gut told my brain to go home, so that's what I did.

The game plan from here would be simple. Get home, get some rest, go for a walk later in the evening, and get to bed early to ensure whatever this event was would pass quickly. I had this mindset going down the elevator. When I reached my car just a few moments later, the panic phase shifted to urgent. My first thought was to call Amy and then my mom, which I did once I got to my car. They both were going about their respective days and actually seemed relatively calm after I struggled vocally to give them the specifics of the last twenty-four hours. My mother, who was an hour away, was on her way toward me immediately. Amy, who had already set off for a business trip to Salt Lake City early that morning, had just deplaned. She could tell that my crippled words became far more dire than the previous day. My fate would be sealed after that call. I fired up my car and bolted for home (which, in hindsight, was a really, really stupid thing to do). There would be no nap or evening walk. Instead, I got home, jumped in the shower, and threw on loose, comfortable clothing knowing that the next destination would be the emergency room at Mount Nittany hospital.

Journal Entry: September 18, 2017 (Afternoon)

This is not to frighten anyone but I'm going to the hospital to get checked out. Something is off! I still feel good for the most part. I have not had any sort of medical complication in years. Perhaps this is just a fluke, perhaps not.

When my mom arrived at my house, she knew within three minutes that something was wrong. The hospital was a quick five-minute drive away. The staff bolted into action immediately after a brief screening. They hooked me up to all sorts of devices, electrodes, and gadgets, all of which I was certainly familiar with by now. One part of this experience was extremely different. The initial sense of panic and fear that I remembered didn't rush over me as IVs were applied to my arms. The staff noticed immediately that I was in control of my surroundings. We were all on the same team here. I had utmost confidence in them. The doctors came in and out of my nook in the ER, calm and collected. They knew that I had been in this sort of position before. Within a few hours, they had me comfortably situated in a room on the ICU unit. All the same smells and sounds burrowed once again into my senses. Only this time I was a little older and a little wiser. There was no doubt that my voice was impacted to some degree. This scared the hell out of me. Being able to still give a firm handshake and retaining my gift of gab were the only tools left in my professional toolbox. Without one or the other, it was pretty fair to assume that my sales career might as well be thrown in a burning dumpster!

Journal Entry: September 19, 2017

I was just informed thirty minutes ago that I was diagnosed with another stroke. This development was in no way tied to the previous incident eleven years ago. It feels like winning the lottery yet being struck by lightning twice type of deals. I have been told that this is a freak event in no way caused by my own doing. The tear was found in my neck causing a clot to pass resulting in the difficulty with speech.

If there is no meaning to all of this, then I am losing my own battle. I do not lose! I'm frustrated beyond belief but towards no one in particular. People will find out in the hours ahead in disbelief. I am relieved that this is not associated with the first go-around. I am not sure as of this moment, yet somehow I wanted it this way. At least I know what the goal is up front and not having to deal with the aftermath later is a slight relief. I'll come back better than ever through all of this. I'll take it and I'll beat it again!

21

GUARANTEED

A hemorrhagic stroke occurs when a weakened blood vessel ruptures. An ischemic stroke occurs when a blood vessel supplying blood to the brain is obstructed. On this day, I found out that I was the owner of both.

So again, for the second time before age forty, I found myself in the confines of a hospital due to yet another acute stroke. As that first night on the floor set in, an intense personal disappointment began to cascade. "I thought that I was supposed to be this upstanding advocate for stroke and traumatic brain injury survivors. Hell, I didn't even realize that one was attacking my body!" Guilt and resentment set in immediately. I pondered in my thoughts. I shouldn't have driven over the last two days, I shouldn't have gone to Lowe's that night, I shouldn't have gone into the office, and furthermore I should have gone to the hospital immediately (Bradley could have driven me). I should have known my body well enough to know that something was extremely off. I should have remembered the F.A.S.T. acronym explaining the major warning signs such as facial drooping, arm weakness, speech difficulty, time to call 911. All of these basic warning signs that I had repeatedly talked about in groups and written about in blogs. This time, I failed myself.

It took one post on outstroken.com and a few phone calls that evening to have all the troops spun into an uproar yet again upon catching word of my condition. My sister Katie immediately drove in from Harrisburg, my friends and employees practically broke down the doors as soon as the green light for visitation was granted. Amy had flown to Salt Lake City that afternoon for meetings, which she cancelled abruptly upon hearing of my situation back East. She connected back via Dallas, then on to Philadelphia, then to State College when a great sense of relief passed over me upon her arrival and initial embrace. Even Christy reached out that evening when she heard and asked if she could be of assistance. As always, I appreciated all the thoughts, prayers, cards, and kind words of encouragement, which once again poured in. The staff of Mount Nittany Medical Center was terrific (for the most part). They all knew that I knew my shit in this department, yet somehow felt the obligation to look after me as one of their own. The on-site physical therapist was quoted as saying, "Dude, I have no position to be of assistance here. On a physical level, you have this stroke thing figured out." The speech pathologist gave me a few pages of tongue twisters to exercise my tongue and mouth muscles, which actually did help, yet for one reason or another she also acknowledged that my stroke expertise was above her pay grade and cleared me immediately.

Let's just say over the next few days that my family would disagree with my speech status. I likely built an illusion that my condition was not as bad as the test results reported back, but in hindsight, my speech was in rough shape. We never saw the speech pathologist again. We contacted friends who were speech pathologists and researched local facilities to find additional resources. In the meantime, we all did tongue twisters together. It became a game of sorts. I'd record myself and watch my progress. I could control what I could control.

The off-site neurologist who took my case was an older man named Dr. Karr. His approach was short, clinical, and scientific. I expected he'd be more personal and maybe even a touch intrigued or impressed by my stroke credentials at my age. After days of tests, including two CT scans and an EKG, which if you had forgotten from the first round measures brain waves to detect and track seizure patterns, we were anxious to hear the results. Once the results were in, Dr. Karr gave us a short, clinical, and scientific explanation that boiled down to not knowing what could have caused this. Hell, seems anyone can cough or sneeze and have the same thing happen. They'd even run genetic tests, but we needed to wait on those results. So, we waited. We waited for an action plan to get me stabilized. We waited for discharge. We waited. And we waited some more.

While we waited, the nurses and staff took great care of me, and all of us. My assigned internist would stop by and give updates. On the afternoon of the fourth day, the internist explained we should be ready to discharge soon, and Dr. Karr would come by to finalize details. My hopes were up. We all had our hopes up.

Then, it all went downhill quickly. Dr. Karr showed up and said I'd be staying another night. He appeared to be in a hurry—par for the course, it seemed. No real reason. No real explanation. I just heard that I was going to have to stay another night. So did Amy. Then, before I knew it, she bolted out of the room. I later learned she had gone to the nurses' station and requested another neurologist. The nurse understood and said she would find someone else to answer the questions we all had. This was not the first time this head nurse had dealt with bedside manner issues.

After searching the roster, we were offered apologies, as Dr. Karr was the only neurologist available. We all agreed that we'd rather ask him our questions than no one, so if he was our choice, we'd at least like the time we originally deserved.

"I hear you have questions," he stated from the doorway. Yes, yes, we did. Why? What was the reason? It turns out insurance wasn't going to pay for the self-administered medication it would require for me to go home now. We asked how much it was. There's a big difference between $200 and $2,000 or even $10,000. Turns out it was closer to the $200 range. Done. For peace of mind and to be able go home, that's not cheap but it's not unreasonable. Regardless, it's certainly not as expensive as another night in the hospital. We expressed that and closed the deal.

Let's just say the point was taken that a medical professional should not make assumptions, but rather inform a patient about his or her options and equip the patient to make well-informed decisions about his or her care. Lesson for all—you have to advocate for yourself. You have to advocate for your loved ones.

Our message was received loud and clear. His bedside manner changed drastically for the remainder of my stay.

All told, I spent a total of five days in the ICU unit of Mount Nittany Medical Center. My positive outlook was still intact. I was calm, while still processing what happened. This second event did shake me for certain though. This setback confirmed what had rattled inside my gut eleven years ago. Once you've had an initial attack to the brain, the possibility of a relapse is always out there. I remember how the fear had set in as they wheeled me out of the hospital the last time that I'd gotten myself into a situation like this. "When I get out, what's going to become of me? Am I going to fall? Am I going to ever walk again? Am I going to have more seizures? Am I going to have another stroke? Am I ever going to live a normal life again?" The twisted irony of it all is that the answer was "Yes" to all of the above.

And now another layer of setback had sunk in. How much of my impacted speech would I get back? At that point, I had no idea. You could definitely tell that there were some components of my speech that were more affected than others. Even in the hospital, some words rolled out of my mouth unaffected, just as they had a week earlier. However, others locked my tongue up something awful for no rhyme or reason. It was as if the brain structured the word, sentence, or phrase perfectly but the signal broke from brain to vocal chords for whatever reason. Now, the positive here was that multiple speech pathologists who evaluated me thereafter said that most of the minor speech disfigurement should return to close to normal with time and practice. "With practice?" Listen, people, if there is one thing that I'm pretty damn good at it is talking! This form of therapy I would excel at! And so I began to craft a "do it yourself" speech therapy syllabus for as long as it would take to get back as much of my voice as possible. I wrote in my journal some of the words that were really hanging me up, such as "science," "precise," "lighter," "about," "ceiling," "paper clip," "celery," "backwards," "lithium," "sure," "tray," "blanket," "ticket," "adequate," "balloon," "rubber," "tornado," "sentence," "impressive," "cadence," and most memorable, the word "cookie." I couldn't get it out. I still don't understand if it was the "k" sound or wrapping my voice around the "oo" sound. I had not a clue. But I could not say the word "cookie" for anything.

At some point toward the end of my hospital stay, an epiphany of sorts started to set in. After my status was downgraded from critical/ acute, the staff started to look at my situation differently. On at least four occasions, professionals (including the neurologist we'd given a verbal beating to three days prior) began dropping by my room with fellow associates to meet me (or "observe my current condition"). The introductions began the same way each time as handshakes and pleasantries were exchanged. "This is the guy that I was telling you about," they all would say almost boastfully of the prized tenant of room 235. My story of what I had been through over the past eleven years was regurgitated multiple times. Even with my newly impacted speech, I did my best to fill in the gaps as best I could. "So, what you're telling me here is that this guy, with this personality and lifestyle, has been impacted by both a hemorrhagic bleed and an ischemic clot and he's not even forty years of age yet? That's nearly impossible! That has the same probability of having been struck by lightning twice! This simply does not happen. It just doesn't." I also heard, "Well, Jonathan, you have one of the most positive outlooks on your situation that we have ever seen. Some people are put on this earth to inspire others. You are one of these people." That was the message expressed each time.

At the end of each one of those interactions, the door would be pulled to a slightly ajar position. I would be left alone in that bed to reflect on all these speeches. One female physical therapist stated jovially after hearing my story that "I have no idea what you do for a living currently, but you should think about becoming a national advocate for this cause. You are some sort of stroke anomaly." Her words really warmed my heart. As I processed her comments, I turned my thoughts inward. Perhaps this stroke deal is my mission. I have been so passionate about the cause for over a decade now. This is the one thing in my life that I feel I'm really, really good at! My talent level on a stage with my voice and guitar, or performance on a tennis court or golf course, or expertise as an avid skier on a snow-covered black diamond trail cannot compete with my knowledge of how to adapt when faced with adversity.

On the day of my discharge I was in awesome spirits. There were no marching bands on-site, no fanfare or speeches needed. I had dodged yet another bullet and become wiser from it. I may have inspired a few individuals during my stay. Upon leaving this time around, I was not nearly as scared as I had been eleven years ago. This was the way a patient should feel when exiting through the front doors and returning to the world, I thought. Typically, with any extended hospital stay, an array of hurdles, roadblocks, differences of opinion, and emotions are going to come into play at certain points. Its all part of the roller-coaster ride—that feeling when you get released back out into the world. The feeling will change you for better or worse (or at least it should). And it goes back to the *Shawshank Redemption* reference when Red says, "Get busy living or get busy dying." That line is so great and so true. I had to once again be hypersensitive to my daily routine. They again put me on a high dose of blood thinners that I had to inject into my abdomen daily.

I reduced my office hours, excessive exercise regimen, salt intake, and alcohol consumption upon doctor's recommendation even though he had no solid evidence as to what had caused a second stroke. Further CT scans and doctor visits were coordinated prior to release as well.

If there is one other thing that I'm extremely good at, it is the gift of gab. It was on me to retrain my voice to communicate effectively. I worked on articulating all of those words that I wrote down in my journal. When there was no one around or while I would be walking on a desolate trail in the evening, I would speak my thoughts out loud as a means to retrain the damaged mouth and throat muscles. I worked hard on the speech therapy aspects each day. And just the same way a guitar player learns a new riff, with time and with practice, the pieces of the puzzle would fuse together to create the desired result. Singing turned out to be a good source of advanced therapy, forcing the focus on voice range as well as phrase articulation. By the time all was said and done, after nearly three months, I managed to get my voice back to roughly 90 percent of normal. Sometimes, at the end of a long day, I can hear my voice begin to slur a little from the minute remains of those impacted muscles. And that is fine by me. I hold the minuscule impairment close as a reminder of the event. And I use the event as another tool in my box knowing that this second attack could have potentially left me in a far worse condition.

22

HERE

I had known the now CEO of Worldwide Express Tom Madine since I attended my basic sales training some sixteen years ago. As a former franchisee, he built one of the top organizations in the system that was used as the backbone infrastructure when Worldwide began its evolution into a direct-operating company a few years back. I have always admired Tom immensely for his accomplishments both on a personal and professional level. He too once had been a young hustler who started his career in a competitive outside sales environment and organically grew from within the organization just as so many of us had. We got to know each other quite well as I made my way through the system and into an ownership role. He always gave me sound advice on the business as well as my personal life. Tom is just a great, humble dude. He's the guy who always treats his employees and colleagues with utmost respect while maintaining the role as a family man as well. He's still got a bit of that youthful and hungry "sales person swagger" and you can tell this by simply watching him work a room. He's a ball buster but takes his share of jabs in a good roasting. And you feel honored to pick his brain for ten minutes at a happy hour over the business or matters otherwise.

Tom reached out to me a few days after he caught word that I was discharged from the hospital and back in the office. We talked for fifteen minutes from my office. He joked at my slurring of words because he knew that I would get a kick out of his typical banter. Before we said our appropriate adieus, he said the following, which led into our last few minutes of conversation, switching from a medical check-in, "We all hope you're on the mend up there," said the CEO grabbing the oximeter for a quick read of pulse: "When you feel the time is right, you give me a call for discussion," he said. To which I replied "Give me a couple weeks to get my affairs in order up here, and I'll be down to talk." I certainly couldn't have predicted that we'd have the conversation on that day due to the weight of the past week's events, yet I did know that the timing felt right. That conversation marked the beginning of my exit strategy from Worldwide Express. It had been a really sweet journey, a truly cool run. In a few short months, this ride would be over.

Now the key question in my situation became—what does the next chapter of Jonathan's life look like? I hadn't a clue. However, here is what I did know; after sixteen years with the same organization—which I adored—I felt that I was slowly starting to lose my ripe passion for the transportation industry. Ultimately, I was trying desperately to hold on to what I'd had. This was the hand that was dealt to me. I needed to stay in the game no matter if I was essentially bluffing or not. No fortune teller could read what the future held for me. But it's fascinating how the entrepreneurial mind works. After my first stroke, I began to lose touch with the industry. At the end of the day, a year-and-a-half recovery period, filled with hospitals, time off, missed corporate trainings, doctor appointments, not to mention adaptation to a far-different-looking world, will do that to

a person. The second stroke simply solidified what had been shifting over those ten years. And as one passion began to fade, another grew stronger. I simply didn't realize it then.

The demand has been there for a very long time. Just jump on to the internet and you'll understand what I'm talking about. You can get on Facebook or Instagram or social media outlet of your choosing and boast to your friends about some fancy restaurant that you're currently at. You can jump on the Uber app and select a vehicle that fits your specifications and will pick you up and whisk you off to a destination of your choosing. You can pay almost any bill online without ever writing a check. You can use Favor to have sushi delivered to your front door. You can even swipe right on Tinder if you want to roll the dice with the opposite sex for an evening when visiting an urban area. But (and I do stress "But"!) how do you fix a major medical setback? What's next? What's the game plan? How do we get you or a loved one back? And, granted, there are certainly websites and blogs and books and publications and gadgets and testimonials. And might I also add that the amount of support has improved as I actively plunge forward in my fourteenth year of recovery. But unfortunately there is a very real fact to face. The resources are growing because the stats are escalating. And this is where the Google machine becomes a valuable resource when pulling stats for stroke affecting the lives of young people (ages forty and below) due to a whole plethora of reasons from smoking to birth control, to complications in utero, and everything in between. The need for more resources is more important than ever, especially for survivors and caregivers, no matter what the setback entails!

I see it often in hospitals and support groups, in the faces of those whose lives are impacted. Life-changing setbacks such as stroke/ CVA, TBI, aneurisms, spinal cord injury, MS, and paralysis all come with their own sets of daily challenges that affect everyone involved. I participate in multiple stroke support groups throughout the country, and the one complaint I hear constantly is that there are simply not enough tools available throughout the many stages of recovery.

And the recovery journey remains constant after dealing with a major life setback, no matter what it looks like. In some way, I think that I was specifically given my set of personal challenges as some convoluted puzzle to figure out and then inspire others around me. Perhaps teach people in need my bag of tricks, you might say. But the main ingredient will always be attitude. A positive attitude will always figure out how to finish the puzzle even if nonconformative measures are taken to complete a task or reach a goal. Hell, I've been doing this sort of jazz all my life anyway. This is simply another way to repurpose my specific way of thinking.

Stroke and traumatic brain injury awareness and advocacy have become my passion. And with passion comes vision. So, I founded a new business venture and foundation around the concept. I took three key words that summarized my story and then gave them a spin to play off of my personality. Enter Stage Left was started in 2017 with a $25,000 budget and no real clue as to how the model would build itself out. What the hell does "Enter Stage Left" signify, you ask? In a typical theater, "stage left" is the viewpoint facing the audience. Well, you, my friends, are my audience in one capacity or another. I needed a stage, or platform, to tell my story and explain my mission. I "entered" into a completely new view of my body and surroundings after my surgery. And "Left," well, "left side impacted" or "this is what I'm left with going forward"—take your pick. Get the picture? My goal is to educate and inspire survivors, caregivers, and professionals on a national and perhaps even global scale one day.

After I sold my business in State College, I had to figure out "Where's next for me?" I had two stipulations: I wanted an urban lifestyle, and the location's climate had to be at least slightly warmer than what I was dealing with up here in the midst of the Appalachians (though the mountains are fabulous during certain times of the year, snow and ice are not my friends). So, in my typical nature, I jumped in my car, hopped on jets, and toured cities all over the East. Philadelphia, New York, Washington DC, Richmond, Raleigh, Charlotte, Savanna, Jacksonville, Ft. Lauderdale, and Miami were points of interest right off the top of my head. I'd spend a few days at a time kicking around, feeling the pulse, while absorbing the urban vibes. The key though, was to find a more centralized point in terms of logistics if I was going to pull this off right. Well, let me tell you that never in a hundred billion years did I think three years ago that I would pick up and move to Dallas, Texas, of all places. However, as I pondered the idea, it all made complete sense.

Journal Entry/outstroken.com Post: February 2, 2018

For 12 years, I've coined February as my personal "Stroke Appreciation Month." And we all know my shenanigans of celebrating and reflecting on the cause and the journey. This month yet again, I shall attempt to push the limits and inspire all of you who have been a part of my recovery.

After my second go-around this past September (an ischemic clot and a completely separate incident from the hemorrhagic bleed as a result of my surgery years ago) the medical establishment agreed unanimously that at my age and degree of life and health, I am a bit of an anomaly. I feel that I've embraced the challenges in recovery and never let personal goals fade due to disabilities handed to me. And at some point between hospitals, therapy, and recovery, I began to embrace the challenge especially when I started to notice that my story inspired those around me . . . survivors, healthcare professionals, and the caregivers whose lives were also impacted by disability and the challenges of loved ones. I'm neither a therapist nor doctor, but I've lived it! And for me to give anyone in my shoes a bit of hope and sound direction is the best feeling I can think of. It drives me to be better physically and mentally and to push on to live a full and enjoyable life.

I had a wonderful run with Worldwide Express for 16 years, which brought with it experience, a degree of success, and some of the best

MAYBE THEY LEFT TOOLS IN MY BRAIN

memories of my life. Certain opportunities have a shelf life, and I decided in December to follow suit and sell my business back to our corporate office in order to focus on my "Passion Project," which has been in the works for almost a full year to this point. With outstroken.com (now over 1,000 followers strong), I feel this is the right time to follow my head and my heart on this path.

I will be relocating to Dallas, Texas, in a couple short weeks to start an organization focusing on Stroke and Traumatic Brain Injury consultation on a national scale with the goal of building a founda- tion. A huge hospital base, logistical travel sense, professional con- nections in the area, and of course, my partner in adventure who has put countless hours of time and knowledge into building this business model out, makes the transition a no-brainer as I see it. I will keep you all updated.

///

23

ELSE

Have you found the satire in it all yet?

For the most part, anyone who walks into a hospital environment in any capacity confronts a depressing situation. We all think of the sights and smells of the sick in these facilities. The sheer thought of pulling into the parking garage makes many people quiver. Well, now I experience the exact opposite emotion when I pass through the automated sliding front doors of a hospital. The entire environment invigorates me! It makes me proud to show off my Left Side Paralysis merit badge while swaggering through the atriums and lobbies and into elevators and down hallways and corridors. Every time I pass a professional, I make an effort to give greetings and a smile if eye contact is met. In here, I'm proud that they notice my left arm not responding to the natural flow of gait while walking, accompanied by my clenched left fist. They all know. And I want

MAYBE THEY LEFT TOOLS IN MY BRAIN

them to know. Every time I look at the directory located by the elevators, I intentionally look for the ICU unit and think, "Maybe there is someone up there that I can help." I enjoy peering into the physical therapy gymnasiums on my way to where I'm heading, envisioning myself approaching a young survivor who has given up on their personal journey to a desired state of recovery. I think about sharing my journey with that person, giving them the practical wisdom from a survivor who, not long ago, was right where they are now. That's the good stuff! That's why I get so energized by becoming involved with these facilities.

I never intended my journey of survival to become downplayed. Nor do I expect to portray myself as the martyr for the cause. It becomes a person's natural reaction, out of human empathy, to feel bad for me when they hear my story. Well, this was how the events were intended to play out, and I wouldn't change any of that for anything.

So, what did I actually lose through all of this, you may ask? Absolutely nothing! Now that I'm forty-one years of age, I doubt that I could be much more satisfied with the quality of life that I currently have. That entrepreneurial drive paired with the logical foresight of educated financial risk constantly pushes me forward. What was lost physically has given me an entire skill set that revolves around perseverance, which I will utilize forever. I firmly believe that my life was never intended to take some stagnant course. Someone up there gave me the tools and attitude to simply do more with a little bit less.

CPSIA information can be obtained
at www.ICGtesting.com
Printed in the USA
BVHW071809300122
62757OBV00001B/13